ABC OF SPORTS MEDICINE

ABC OF SPORTS MEDICINE

edited by

GREG McLATCHIE

Visiting professor of sports medicine and surgical sciences, University of Sunderland
Consultant surgeon at Hartlepool General Hospital, and
Director of the National Sports Medicine Institute, London

MARK HARRIES

Consultant physician at Northwick Park Hospital, Harrow, and Director of clinical services,
British Olympic Medical Centre, Harrow

CLYDE WILLIAMS

Professor of sport and exercise science,
University of Loughborough

J B KING

Director of the academic department of sports medicine,
London Hospital Medical College
Consultant orthopaedic surgeon, Royal London Hospital, and
Chairman of the British Association of Sport and Medicine

with contributions from

RICHARD BUDGETT, SUE CAMPBELL, ROSLYN CARBON, J C CHAWLA, DAVID A COWAN,
SUSIE DINAN, J D M DOUGLAS, P H FENTEM, J F GOODWIN, JAMES GRAHAM,
VIVIAN GRISOGONO, ROGER G HACKNEY, W S HILLIS, BRYAN JENNETT,
LESLIE KLENERMAN, EVAN L LLOYD, J MACLEAN, DONALD A D MACLEOD,
P D McINTYRE, W J McKENNA, NANETTE MUTRIE, J C M SHARP, PETER N SPERRYN,
D S TUNSTALL-PEDOE, ROGER L WOLMAN, ARCHIE YOUNG

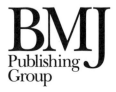

BMJ
Publishing
Group

© BMJ Publishing Group 1995

All rights reserved. No part of this publication may be reproduced, stored in a retrieval system, or transmitted, in any form or by any means, electronic, mechanical, photocopying, recording and/or otherwise, without the prior written permission of the publishers.

First published in 1995
by the BMJ Publishing Group, BMA House, Tavistock Square,
London WC1H 9JR

Second impression 1997
Third impression 1998
Fourth impression 1999

British Library Cataloguing in Publication Data

A catalogue record for this book is available
from the British Library

ISBN 0-7279-0844-8

Typeset by Bedford Typesetters Ltd, and printed and bound by
Craft Print, Singapore

Contents

PREFACE

Participation in sport and exercise has become increasingly popular. Although many more men than women participate, there is some evidence that the gap is closing. The reasons for this increase in participation is an awareness that regular exercise is associated with good health. As living standards improve and leisure time increases so more people have the opportunity to take part in sport. With the continuing reduction of the hours worked per week and the prospect of earlier retirement this trend will probably continue. In schools, too, the reintroduction of team games implies that the exercise habit will become implanted at the earliest age.

In parallel with health benefits there are also risks in sport. Soft tissue injuries constitute a significant part of the workload of doctors who treat sportsmen and sportswomen. This problem is so extensive that it has been described as an "unthwarted epidemic" by some authorities in the United States. Doctors are also asked for advice on diet, travel and immunisations, permitted medication, and medical problems in sport.

Against this background we have invited specialists from many areas of sports medicine and exercise science to present their experience. Our aim is to increase the general understanding of doctors who have an interest in sports medicine but who do not consider themselves specialists. There are now many courses available in sports medicine and exercise science, and the recent initiative of the medical colleges of the United Kingdom of establishing an intercollegiate faculty of sports medicine does imply that training sports medicine is being taken seriously.

Greg McLatchie
Mark Harries
Clyde Williams
John King

May 1995

NATURE, PREVENTION, AND MANAGEMENT OF INJURY

Roger G Hackney

Nature of injury

Intrinsic factors in the causation of injuries

- Age, sex, body weight and composition, and muscle power (for example, imbalance of agonist versus antagonist)
- Muscle stiffness or weakness
- Congenital joint hyperlaxity or conversely poor flexibility
- Malalignment—for example, forefoot varus, hyperpronation, pes cavus, tibia vara, patella baja/alta, genu varum/valgum, femoral anteversion leg length discrepancy, etc

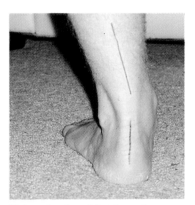

Valgus heel and flat foot of overpronation.

Extrinsic factors in the causation of injuries

- Training methods and competition (high volume and increase in intensity of training, sudden changes in training method, poorly designed training techniques, ineffective rules of the sport, violent play, or ill-timed contact)
- Surfaces (change from running on grass to synthetic track, increased incidence of anterior cruciate ligament injuries on synthetic grass)
- Equipment (power footwear, old or unsuitable training shoes, poorly adjusted bindings on ski-boots, heavy wet footballs, poor landing surfaces for jumpers)
- Environment (cold weather with inadequate warm up leads to reduced elasticity and stiffness, hot and humid weather can cause heat stroke, competing or training in poor light can cause injury)

Unfortunately, injury is inevitable for some of those who participate in sporting activity. Injuries may occur as a result of an acute episode of trauma, such as a fractured tibia in a footballer. Overuse injuries are caused by repeated episodes of microtrauma that individually are insufficient to give rise to macroscopic injury. When healing mechanisms are overcome, however, the end result can be as serious as a fractured neck of femur from a completed stress fracture. The nature of the injury depends on many interrelated elements, but they can be divided into those caused by intrinsic and those caused by extrinsic factors.

Intrinsic factors are concerned with the makeup of the individual person. Preparation and training can alter some of these constituents, which should always be considered in the management of individual people.

Extrinsic factors in injury are those derived from external forces. These range from a clumsy tackle inflicting a sudden violent force on a limb to footwear and the surface being used.

Sport specificity of injury

The injuries suffered by athletes do not differ greatly from those occurring in any other group of people. However, every sport has its own group of injuries that are, to a greater or lesser extent, specific to that sport itself. This has important ramifications when managing an injury, but also in preventing the injury in the first instance. Doctors caring for athletes must have a knowledge of the type and techniques of training involved for a sport and the physiological basis of the type of exercise as well as being familiar with the aspects of competition. Only then can they gain the confidence of their athletes and become closely involved in their return to sport.

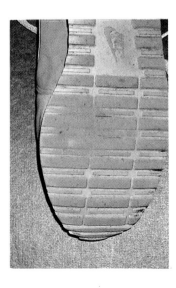

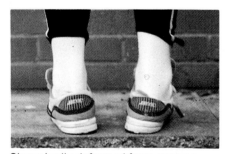

Shoes badly deformed from overuse.

Sole of shoe worn away (50% of shock absorbency lost after 500 miles, about a month's training for a marathon runner).

Prevention of injury

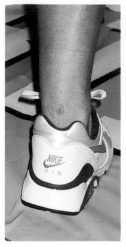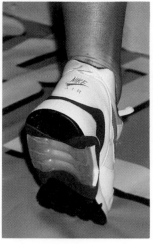

Simple measures in injury prevention: removing from poorly designed shoes heel tabs that impinge on the Achilles tendon, aggravating Achilles tendonitis.

Preventing sports injuries

Intrinsic factors
- Adequate warm up before participation
- Correct stretching techniques
- Strengthening exercises to achieve a balance of muscle power
- Fitness for sport, particularly aerobic—that is, cardiovascular and respiratory fitness, muscle power, and sport specific fitness
- Good nutritional status

Extrinsic factors
- Correct use of equipment, especially footwear
- Avoiding abrupt changes in training methods, effort, and intensity
- Paying due attention to the environment
- Awareness of the second injury syndrome
- Playing within the rules of the sport

Management of injury

Stages of managing a sporting injury

(1) First aid measures

(2) RICE—Rest the injured part, not the rest of the athlete
  Ice, pain relief, and prevention of bleeding
  Compression to reduce swelling
  Elevation of injured part

(3) Early management—make a diagnosis with appropriate investigation and formulate a treatment plan

(4) Maintain cardiovascular and respiratory fitness, while resting the injured part

(5) Strengthening and stretching exercises

(6) Sport specific fitness

(7) Attention to technique, equipment, etc

(8) Competition—staged return by setting targets to achieve simulation of potential areas of risk

---

Preparation

Preparation is the key word when considering prevention of sporting injury. There are very few circumstances in which inadequate preparation cannot be blamed for injury. Training errors cause injury. A footballer with a broken tibia may have been suffering from fatigue because of poor aerobic fitness or may have become a victim of the second injury syndrome—in this case a previous minor knock may have lead to clumsy timing or poor commitment in a tackle.

Victims of overuse injuries have failed to manage correctly their training schedules or have paid inadequate attention to correct use of equipment. A typical example is a runner who uses the same pair of shoes for over a year. After this amount of time the shock absorbency of the shoe is severely reduced and the shoe is deformed, which exaggerates any biomechanical abnormality of the runner and leads to an overuse injury.

Safety equipment

Many sports use safety quipment routinely. Perhaps the most striking example of this is American football, where the more obvious padding covers many yards of taping, strapping, and bracing for added protection. Correct use of such equipment is essential in avoiding injury. The design of helmets has altered and improved to prevent serious neck and face injuries in sports such as icehockey and American football. The simple addition of a harness to prevent falls while jumping has reduced head and neck injury rates in horse riders. When equipment is used it must be maintained and adjusted properly. Unless correctly tuned, ski-boot bindings will prevent the ski from detaching in a fall and lead to knee ligament injury.

Rules of sport

One of the impacts of sports medicine has been in changing the rules of some sports. This rarely occurs by presidential decree, as it did in American football, but in rugby the alteration of scrummaging rules has been brought about to prevent injury. There is now an important medicolegal aspect in terms of adhering to the rules. When considering the intrinsic and extrinsic causes of injury listed earlier, preparation for sport includes several considerations.

Managing a sporting injury is not simply a matter of treating the injured part. A runner who returns to pounding the roads in the same pair of old, worn shoes after his Achilles tendonitis has settled with treatment will relapse without fail. The same principle applies to tennis players with lateral epicondylitis who have not given themselves time to adjust to their new rackets. (It is also necessary to remember that the aim of treatment is a return to sport.)

History

It is imperative that the sporting cause of the injury is discovered. This occasionally requires an intimate knowledge of the sport itself so that a full sporting history can be obtained. However, patients are often able to provide the reasons for their injuries. Liaison with the coach may be invaluable.

Diagnosis

As with the rest of medicine, it is essential to make a diagnosis when managing a sporting injury. Appropriate investigations should be made. Ultrasound scans are particularly useful in this specialty, although the high resolution probes for visualising subcutaneous structures are expensive.

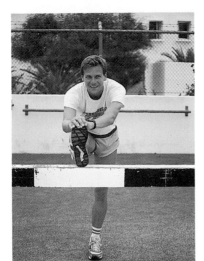

Demonstration of stretching technique

Rehabilitation

Many injuries are caused by premature return to competition before the athlete is ready. The rehabilitation of athletes through all the stages of their return to competition is an integral part of managing the injury.

Athletes often complain that they are simply told to rest and given no more advice. Doctors may complain that athletes seek multiple opinions in order to receive the answers that they want to hear, and not what is best for them. This breakdown in communication can be avoided by the doctor explaining the nature of the injury and emphasising what the athlete should be doing to retain power and fitness. A positive attitude towards rehabilitation should be adopted on both sides. The injury should not be thought of as time lost, but an opportunity to correct some of the deficiencies of those intrinsic factors listed earlier. In addition, athletes may need to be seen by appropriate specialists to investigate chronic fatigue from overtraining, amenorrhoea resulting in stress fractures, or the management of eating disorders.

Drugs

Non steroidal anti-inflammatory agents can be used for analgesia and helping during recovery, but should not be used to mask chronic injury. The non-steroidal anti-inflammatory gels have their uses in sports medicine. In addition to their therapeutic effects they are useful for self massage. Local anaesthetic injections, alone or with corticosteroid, have both diagnostic and therapeutic uses. Although the published evidence is equivocal, injection of corticosteroid around the Achilles tendon should be avoided because of the risk of rupture.

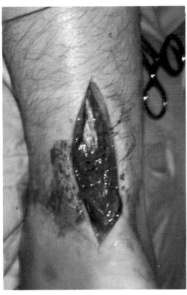

Ruptured Achilles tendon.

Surgery

Surgery has an important role in the management of sports trauma, but the surgeon should ensure that conservative measures, using the principles outlined in this article, have been thoroughly applied.

Physiotherapy

Medical advice is often combined with physiotherapy. Although stretching techniques can be demonstrated in the surgery, supervision by a physiotherapist is recommended. There are many ways athletes will delude themselves that they are stretching adequately.

Physiotherapists will also use massage, friction, faradism, strapping, stretching, and strengthening techniques with manipulation and mobilisations. They may also aid in making a diagnosis with their own techniques, and close working relationships between doctors and physiotherapists are helpful.

Physiotherapy includes the use of electrical treatments such as ultrasound; interferential, short wave diathermy; and laser therapy. Although some basic research work has shown why ultrasound and laser may be effective, they are no substitutes for active "hands on" work.

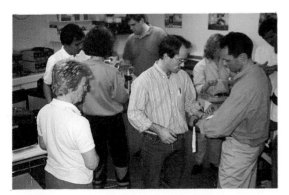

Doctors and physiotherapists perfecting strapping techniques on a British Association of Sport and Medicine course.

Insoles

The use of insoles to modify running gait, after video analysis of running on a treadmill, is becoming increasingly common in the commercial world of sports injury medicine. The results can be dramatic in the treatment of a surprisingly wide variety of conditions. Perhaps the most notable results are in the treatment of medial periostitis of the tibia in runners. Unfortunately, the use of insoles has become excessive and uncontrolled.

Conclusion

Important factors in managing sporting injury

Prevention (general fitness, training regimen, equipment use)

Management

- History to establish cause(s) of injury and thus make correct diagnosis and prevent recurrence
- Examination (of athlete and equipment)
- Investigation
- Diagnosis—for correct treatment
- Treatment appropriate to injury (rest, drugs, physiotherapy, surgery)
- Maintenance of general fitness (of uninjured parts)
- Correction of poor training programmes
- Rehabilitation—gradual, structured regimen
- Emphasis of importance of warm up before, stretch after, exercise
- Prevention of too early return to sport—to avoid recurrence of second injury

Management of a sporting injury requires an assessment of why the injury occurred, treating the injury itself while maintaining fitness, and a gradual structured rehabilitation programme through to competition. Breakdown can occur at any stage along the path of return to sport. Doctors should liase with the athlete's coach to alter bad training regimens and check the sporting history for other factors contributing to the risk of injury.

Athletes are enthusiastic and rewarding patients to treat. The British Association of Sport and Medicine runs an educational programme covering all aspects of sports medicine. Anyone interested should contact the author.

HEAD INJURY

Greg McLatchie, Bryan Jennett

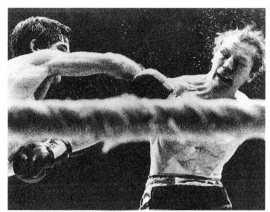

In boxing injuries to the head account for 40% of all injuries. A boxer who sustains three knockouts is not permitted to fight for the rest of the season.

Most sports related injuries are musculoskeletal, affecting limbs or trunk, and related to specific risks associated with particular sports. Head injuries by contrast can occur in many sports and, except those incurred during boxing, are accidental. Unlike other injuries, the effects of which are usually maximal at onset, injury to the head may precipitate a process of intracranial disorder that can convert a mild initial injury into a life threatening condition from secondary complications. Moreover, even mild injuries are often associated with considerable temporary disability, and repeated mild injuries can result in cumulative brain damage. Doctors on sports fields have to decide whether patients with head injury can resume play or, if not, what further immediate management is needed and when they can play again. The answers to these questions depend on a sensible balancing of risks.

Nature of damage to the brain

Incidence of sporting head injuries in Glasgow requiring neurosurgical admission	
Golf	28%
Horse riding	16%
Football	14%
Shooting	10%
Climbing	8%
Rugby	6%
Boxing	4%

Source: Lindsay KW, McLatchie GR, Jennett.B. Serious head injury in sport. *BMJ* 1980;**281**:789-91.

Intracranial haematomas
- *Extradural*—usually related to bleeding from middle meningeal vessels in the temporal or temporoparietal regions
- *Intradural*
  Subdural—usually caused by bleeding from superficial veins ruptured indirectly by shearing forces or directly by impact
  Intracerebral—most commonly occurring in the frontal and temporal lobes, and usually associated with immediate impairment of consciousness as a result of associated diffuse injury of white matter
- *Subarachnoid haemorrhage*
- *Mixed types*

It is damage to the brain that matters when the head is hit. Injuries to the scalp or skull are important only as indicators of the possibility of underlying impact damage or of the risk of complications that could cause secondary brain damage. Either impact or secondary brain damage may be diffuse or focal, and this will influence the clinical features.

Primary brain damage

Impact (or primary) damage can take two forms:

(1) *Cerebral contusions*—Bruising on the brain surface due to the brain's impact with the overlying skull—are the commonest form of impact damage. Contusion may be focal underneath a fracture resulting from a focal impact, blunt or penetrating, or it may be diffuse, resulting from the brain as a whole being thrown against the rough interior surface of the skull and dural dividers. Diffuse contusion results when the head as a whole decelerates, usually by hitting the ground, in which case the contusions are usually bilateral, affecting the tips of both frontal and temporal poles regardless of where the head was actually struck. Contusions themselves do not necessarily cause impaired consciousness or focal neurological signs (unless they are over the motor strip, the speech area, or the visual cortex). Their main importance is that they may initiate secondary local brain swelling, and continued bleeding may produce an intradural haematoma.

(2) *Diffuse axonal injury*—Widespread tearing of the white matter fibres in the subcortical areas of the brain. This can occur without pronounced contusions or a fracture of the skull, and it usually causes immediate unconsciousness.

Secondary brain damage

Secondary brain damage results from three main mechanisms:

(1) Raised intracranial pressure results from either an acute intracranial haematoma or brain swelling, often both. Acute intracranial haematomas may be extradural or intradural. If intradural they may be either subdural or intracerebral but are often a combination of both—forming the so called burst lobe, usually located frontotemporally. A haematoma causes midline shift of the brain with

Head injury

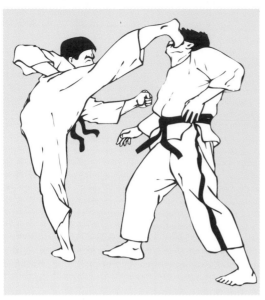

An uncontrolled (illegal) roundhouse kick to the head.

a tentorial hernia causing distortion of the brain stem, where secondary haemorrhage eventually spells a fatal outcome. *Brain swelling* is a consequence of vascular engorgement or cerebral oedema, or both, and it may be focal or diffuse. Respiratory obstruction or inadequacy (causing a raised $Paco_2$ and lowered Pao_2) will cause vasodilatation in cerebral vessels and subsequent engorgement in the brain as a whole, but also aggravates any focal swelling around contusions. Oedema of the hemisphere often occurs after surgical removal of an acute intracranial haematoma, especially if this has been delayed.

(2) *Hypoxia and ischaemia* are found in a high proportion of fatal cases of brain damage and contribute considerably to disability in survivors of severe injuries. The main cause is raised intracranial pressure, which reduces the flow of blood into the skull, but an aggravating factor is lowered blood pressure and haemoglobin content in the blood because of associated extracranial injuries. These are likely to occur in sporting injuries only when the whole body has suffered violence, as in accidents associated with climbing, horse riding, and racing cars or motorcycles.

(3) *Intracranial infection (meningitis or brain abscess)* is a possibility when the dura has been penetrated by injury. Compound depressed fracture of the vault can introduce contamination direct into the intracranial cavity, whereas a fractured base of skull can put the intracranial cavity into contact with the nasal sinuses or the middle ear cavity.

Clinical features and action required

The Glasgow coma score	
Eye opening	
Spontaneous	4
To voice	3
To pain	2
None	1
Best verbal response	
Orientated	5
Confused	4
Inappropriate words	3
Incomprehensible	2
None	1
Best motor response	
Obeys commands	6
Localises pain	5
Withdraws from pain	4
Flexes to pain	3
Extends to pain	2
None	1
Possible total (range)	3-15

Neurological history
This will be obtained from the doctor's own observations, witnesses, the ambulance crew, or other emergency service staff
1 What were the circumstances of the accident? (tackle, scrum collapse, fall, etc)
2 Has the patient talked at any time?
3 What was the patient's Glasgow coma score at the accident scene?
4 Has the patient's Glasgow coma score altered en route?
5 Has the patient taken alcohol or any other drugs?
6 Has the patient had a fit?

Altered consciousness

Altered consciousness is the hallmark of diffuse brain damage. It is evidenced by immediate change in responsiveness and in subsequent loss of memory for an interval after injury—post-traumatic amnesia (PTA). The Glasgow coma scale is now the accepted means of assessing patients with head injuries, both initially and for continued observations, for signs of deterioration that would indicate complications that call for immediate action. Most head injuries are mild, resulting in only a minute or so of eyes closed coma with no speech and not obeying commands. As a player regains consciousness the important observation is whether there is a rapid return to full orientation (in person, time, and place). All who have been completely knocked out, and some who have been only dazed, will have a period of incomplete recovery, during which automatic behaviour may enable them to continue playing but of which period they have no subsequent memory. When there has been a definite period of coma, the post-traumatic amnesia always extends for a considerable time after return to responsive behaviour, and the duration of the amnesia is considered the best guide to the severity of diffuse brain damage. A study of 544 rugby footballers in Britain some years ago found 56% had suffered at least one head injury associated with post-traumatic amnesia; this had lasted more than an hour in 58 players, of whom only 38 had been admitted to hospital for observation.

Field assessment of players with head injury

Scalp wounds often lead to brisk bleeding, and players should be removed for careful inspection of the wound and control of haemorrhage. Such players are not permitted to stay on the field because of the risk of transmitting HIV. The wound may then be assessed with a sterile gloved finger to assess whether there is a fracture. This is often easier to feel than see. Patients with compound depressed fractures of the vault suffer only local brain damage and, as they often do not lose consciousness, the potential seriousness of the injury can easily be overlooked. Scalp wounds in sport are most commonly the result of being struck by a golf club or ball, billiards cue, bat, or racket. If there is evident herniation of brain tissue through the skull the wound should be covered with a dressing soaked in sterile saline and immediate transport for neurological care or advice arranged. Patients with suspected fractures should firstly have bleeding controlled by closing the scalp with through and through interrupted sutures before transport to hospital. Minor cuts, however, can be sutured with 2/0 or 3/0 silk and, provided that the wound can be covered, the player may return to the field if fully conscious.

Field assessment of level of consciousness

Neurological examination

- Glasgow coma scale
- Pupil sizes and responses to light
- Examination of ears and nose for blood, cerebrospinal fluid, haemotympanum
- Sensation (including the perianal area)
- Deep tendon reflexes (including plantar responses)

The doctor should have witnessed the incident and when called on to the field by the referee should ask the player appropriate questions like: "What happened to you?", "What is the score?", "Where are you?", etc. If the doctor knows the player well then questions relating to family, home, or possessions may indicate whether confusion is present. Eye opening and pupillary size and response to light can also be observed at this initial assessment.

Some field tests, such as finger to nose, finger to finger, or asking the patient to move certain limbs, may assess the best motor response. Equilibrium is often impaired after concussion. Heel to toe standing with the eyes open or closed is not possible in 35% of such players, and standing on one foot with the other suspended is not possible in 50% (the foot on the ground moves or the suspended foot touches the ground). Unfortunately, false positive results also occur, but these tests may indicate the need for more detailed examination in the medical room.

If a player has not lost consciousness and has full memory of the event he or she may continue to play. It should, however, be a rule to send off any player who does not immediately regain full consciousness and orientation. Players with post-traumatic amnesia are at risk of further injury if allowed to play on because their automatic behaviour may not allow them to protect themselves as efficiently as they normally would.

A more difficult decision to make is what further management players or contestants with head injury need. They should be referred to hospital if they are still confused or worse after 10 minutes or so. That would also apply to those in whom an open injury is suspected because of a scalp laceration or blood and fluid coming from the nose or ears. The accident and emergency department can then decide whether a skull *x* ray is required to exclude a skull fracture.

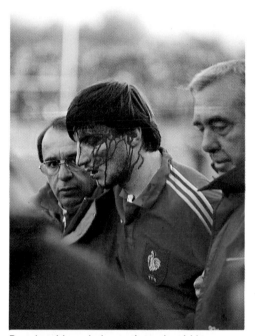

People with scalp lacerations should be referred to hospital for radiology for possible skull fracture.

If a vault fracture is found then the patient will need to be kept in for observation, and probably computed tomography, because the risk of an *acute intracranial haematoma* is considerably increased if there is a vault fracture. Over half the patients with acute intracranial haematomas requiring surgery had been walking and talking when first seen at hospital, and some 15% had remained fully orientated ever since their accident. Delay in recognising and removing an acute intracranial haematoma is the commonest cause of avoidable mortality and morbidity after head injury. In sports medicine it is therefore important to ensure that any player with head injury who goes home from an away or a home game is continuously accompanied by a colleague who can observe whether there is any change in level of consciousness (for example, becoming confused), complaints of increasing headache, or vomiting. Family and friends should be informed of the need to maintain this observation. The occurrence of any of these features calls for immediate referral to hospital (even if the player has already been seen and discharged from hospital).

Head injury card

This patient has received an injury to the head. A careful examination has been made and no sign of any serious complications has been found.

It is expected that recovery will be rapid, but in such cases it is not possible to be quite certain.

If you notice any change of behaviour, vomiting, dizziness, headache, double vision, excessive drowsiness, please telephone the hospital at once.

No alcohol.   No analgesics.   No driving.

Accident and emergency departments sending home patients with head injury now usually give the family or accompanying people a head injury card with these instructions. Sports organisations might make use of such a card, which will include the telephone number of the local hospital. Players who have sustained head injury should avoid alcohol for at least the next 24 hours because they will probably be unduly susceptible to it and also because its effects may lead to confusion in interpreting symptoms that could indicate complications.

After more severe injuries the possibility of *extracranial injuries* should always be considered, because these are easily overlooked in comatose patients who cannot draw attention to them. Cervical spine fractures, chest and abdominal injuries, as well as limb fractures all need to be looked for. Suspected cervical spine fractures require

Head injury

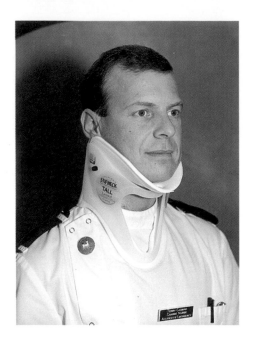

splintage initially with manual in-line stabilisation with the patient supine and the head in the neutral position. The attendant grasps the mastoid processes and a semi rigid collar can then be applied (for example, the Philadelphia/Stifneck). Unconscious patients to be transported from the scene of injury require care to avoid airway obstruction; they should be put in the semiprone coma position until paramedics arrive and can institute suction and intubation. If intubation is required an assistant grasps the mastoid processes and the front of the semi-rigid collar can then be safely removed as it can impede mouth opening and does not contribute significantly to neck stabilisation during laryngoscopy. Manual in-line stabilisation reduces neck movement during intubation but care must be taken to avoid excessive axial traction, which may cause distraction or subluxation. Ideally three or four people are required: the first pre-oxygenates and intubates, the second applies cricoid pressure, the third maintains cervical stabilisation and the fourth, if present, can give intravenous drugs and assist. Both nasotracheal and orotracheal intubation are given equal emphasis when dealing with patients with suspected cervical spine injury who are unconscious. The use of anaesthetic induction agents and neuromuscular blockers may be given in relation to the experience of the attending physician or paramedic. Nasotracheal intubation in a conscious patient is contraindicated if a basal skull fracture is suspected or if there is a risk of causing epistaxis, vomiting, or regurgitation.

Sequelae of head injuries

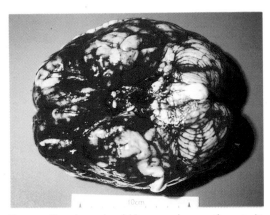

Traumatic subarachnoid haemorrhage—the result of an uncontrolled karate roundhouse kick.

Injuries that were severe, either initially or because of complications, are often associated with persisting, even permanent effects. Changes in mental function are the most consistent, and also the most disabling. These include loss of intellectual capacity, poor recent memory, and personality change. Physical sequelae include hemiparesis, dysphasia, hemianopia, cranial nerve palsies, and traumatic epilepsy.

Mild injuries commonly cause considerable disability for 2-3 weeks. Patients report headaches and dizziness, lack of concentration, fatigue, and difficulties in coping with high level mental functions. These symptoms were once believed to be largely psychological, perhaps motivated by claims for liability, and rare in athletes. Psychometric tests, however, have now shown clear evidence of impaired information processing for 2-3 weeks after injury. Moreover, athletes often suffer from these symptoms after concussion, although they are less common after severe injury, perhaps because they are expected less in the early stages of injury. It is therefore important to ensure that players with head injury take time off work but are reassured that these symptoms are expected to be temporary and do not forecast any continuing disability.

Return to sport

> ### Recommended periods of rest from play or training in contact sports
> - For a memory deficit <2 minutes—at least 48 hours
> - For loss of consciousness or post-traumatic amnesia >2 minutes—15 days
> - For severe concussion (≥3 minutes loss of consciousness)—a month

All participants in contact sports should be required to take three weeks off the sport after a definite head injury and longer if still suffering symptoms after concussion. There is good evidence that a second injury has a greater effect than an initial one and that repeated injuries, even if mild, can cause cumulative damage. For boxers and horse riders, who are most at risk of repeated injury, there must come a time when retirement is recommended for those injured often. Players of contact sports who have had a craniotomy should probably not play again, as the bone flap can be at risk of displacement.

Details relating to head injury incidents must be recorded in either the club's accident book or the fighter's personal record book. In combat sports like boxing the rest time after a knockout is four weeks. Fighters who are knocked out more than three times a year are suspended for the rest of the season.

Prevention of head injury

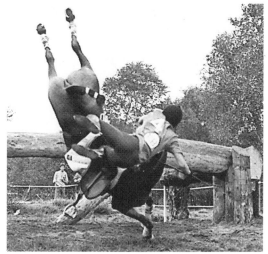

In horse riding hats approved to BSI standards must be worn. Multiple injuries can result from falls like this.

Prevention of primary head injury should be the aim, but in some sports like boxing this would be extremely difficult to achieve unless there were radical changes in the rules. In non-combative sports, however, most injuries are accidental. In some—such as skateboarding, cycling (that is, leisure cycling in children), horse riding, and climbing—head injury can be anticipated and protective headgear should be worn. The age range of youngsters injured while playing golf (from under 16 in one study) suggests that they should be forewarned of the need to stand well clear when others are wielding golf clubs.

Sports that make use of headgear are increasing in number—American football, winter sports, cricket, climbing, cycling, skateboarding, aerial sports, etc. The value of protective headgear in motorcycle and autosport racing accidents has been well established and in sports like steeple chase riding primary serious head injury and cumulative damage have been reduced after these risks were identified. The helmet design used by these jockeys resembles that of a motor cycle crash helmet. The Pony Club compels competing riders to wear an approved jockey skull cap (BS4472) or a riding hat with a flexible peak (BS6473). Stable lads are not insured unless they wear ND4472 type caps, and a change in attitude towards the use of these by the three million people who ride for pleasure would probably reduce the high incidence of head injuries sustained in riding accidents. Although legislation now compels young equestrians to wear proper protective headgear, fashion is more likely to persuade them to do so. The Young Riders Protective Headgear Act 1990 requires children of 14 and under to wear an approved hat, suitably harnessed, when riding on the highway.

During boxing training sessions head protection is regularly worn and is now a feature of the Olympic Games. In countries where headgear is compulsory there has been a reduction in the number of facial cuts and knockouts. Controlling the type of sparring and limiting the number of fights in a boxer's career has been suggested to reduce the risk of cumulative damage. In one survey the risk increased after 40 fights. In addition, the use of padded or sprung flooring protects against serious injury in combat sports.

Prevention of secondary brain damage depends on recognising the risks of certain types of injury and ensuring that medical aid is sought. Some sporting events are attended by a doctor but in many the referee or trainer must learn what to do. Education in this topic is currently being addressed by the National Coaching Foundation and supported by many of the governing bodies of sport.

The photograph of the riding accident was taken by John Lloyd Parry, that of the boxing match is from George Outram Newspapers, and that of the injured rugby player is reproduced with permission of Colorsport. The head injury card is adapted from: Pemberton D. Acute head injuries in sport. *Int J Sports Med* 1992;4:12-3.

Summary of clinical features and action required

Head injury
- Not knocked out
- Knocked out

Not knocked out:
- No amnesia
- Alert
- Orientated
- No neurological deficit

→ May play on

Knocked out:
- Amnesia
- Drowsiness
- Disorientated
- Neurological deficit

→ Removal from event and observe

- Improvement to full recovery → Give head injury instructions and send home under supervision
- Persistent unconsciousness Disorientation Any neurological signs → Refer to hospital Further investigation and admission probable

MANAGEMENT OF THE ACUTELY INJURED JOINT

J B King

Diagnosis

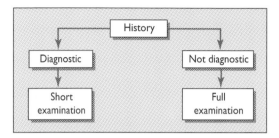

Far too often treatment of injuries to major joints starts without a diagnosis being made.

History

In acute joint injury it may not always be possible to get a good history—for example, when a scrum has collapsed. In many cases, however, the story points to the eventual diagnosis. A fall on the point of the shoulder damages the acromioclavicular or sternoclavicular joint; a rugby tackle that knocks the leading arm into external rotation while abducted 90° indicates a shoulder dislocation; the non-contact twisting deceleration injury of the knee followed by a snapping or popping sensation and rapid swelling is usually associated with a torn anterior cruciate. So a history really is important and is well worth the time spent before the physical examination.

Examination

Look at the joint—Appreciable swelling will be apparent immediately, and deformity (such as patella dislocation) should not be missed. The step deformity of subluxed or dislocated acromioclavicular joints should be obvious, as would be the more subtle sharpening of the point of the shoulder when that joint is dislocated.

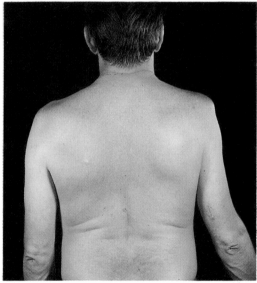

Dislocated right shoulder. Note the prominence of the tip of the acromium with a dent below it, rather than a normal deltoid profile.

Feel the joint—The first thing to feel for is the tenderness, which is the marker of localised injury. Look at patients' faces for apprehension when you first touch them, because once you have hurt them you are going to lose their cooperation. It is essential to feel the landmark points around a particular joint. Using the ankle as an example, gentle but specific palpation over the swollen lateral structures will differentiate the tenderness of the fibula itself if it is fractured from the tenderness overlying the anterior component of the lateral ligament, which runs almost horizontally forward from the tip of the fibula and is far more often injured. In the knee it is important to remember that the lower end of the medial collateral ligament inserts some 10 cm below the joint line and if you do not feel here you miss sprains of this ligament. Bone contours can be palpated, and this is particularly useful at the elbow, where the loss of the triangular relation between the olecranon and the medial and lateral epicondyles is an indicator of a dislocation. At the shoulder the relation between the front of the humeral head and the coracoid process is altered in dislocations, and a palpable step deformity can be felt in severe lesions of the sternoclavicular joint.

Move the joint—There is no need to assess much active movement other than to establish whether or not the joint can move. This will detect lesions such as a tear of the extensor apparatus of the knee or the rotator cuff in the shoulder.

When passive movement is restricted, however, it is necessary to decide whether this is because of pain from muscle spasm, because the joint itself is not in the normal position (that is, is dislocated), or because something within the joint is blocking the movement (locked knee, which means lack of full extension). The decision depending on how soon after an acute injury a patient is examined. A club doctor on the touchline is able to assess the joint before the painful muscle spasm has set in and stopped it moving. For the next few days it is very difficult to distinguish between muscle spasm, dislocation, and a locked joint, and it may well only be possible again a fortnight or so after the injury.

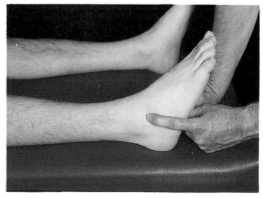

Palpation of the anterior component of lateral ligament of ankle.

Stages before reaching diagnoses

- History of how the injury was sustained
- Examination:
  Look for swelling, bruising, skin lesions, bone deformity
  Feel for tenderness (bone or ligament), bone contours, relations between bones, or deformity
  Move the joint (check particularly for passive and abnormal movement)
- Investigations:
  Aspiration for blood (haemarthrosis)
  Radiology (plain, ultrasound scanning)
- Diagnosis:
  Differential and favoured

Look for abnormal movement—Using the knee as an example, check for abnormal opening of the inner or outer side when stress is applied. The posterior structures are rarely injured and can maintain stability in the fully straightened knee. They should therefore be relaxed by bending the knee to about 30°C. A valgus or varus force can then be applied (while the leg is prevented from rotating) to establish whether the collateral ligaments have been torn. In this same position the femur can be stabilised in one hand and the tibia gently pulled forward and pushed back with the other. This is perhaps the easiest test of the integrity of the anterior cruciate ligament.

Investigation

Aspiration—If the patient is in the surgery and has an acutely swollen joint (usually the knee) the joint should be aspirated to see whether there is blood in it because, in the knee, about three quarters of acute haemarthroses indicate a torn anterior cruciate. The aspiration technique is simple; with clean hands simply clean the skin with standard solution, then introduce a light blue needle above the superolateral aspect of the patella through all the structures, pointing to the back of the mid-point of the patella. This will enter the joint and you can then aspirate. This is not a therapeutic aspiration; you need to get 1 cm³ or so into the syringe just to be sure that it is a genuine haemarthrosis and not a little blood from the perforated soft tissues. I have never seen subsequent infection in an aspirated joint of a patient who did not have some risk factor such as immunosuppression, diabetes, or a skin lesion at the site of the needle puncture. If aspiration does show blood in the joint the patient must be urgently evaluated in hospital. Drawing some air into the syringe, however, and rotating the syringe to coat its walls with the blood will show whether there are any fat globules in the film in which case there is an intra-articular fracture as well.

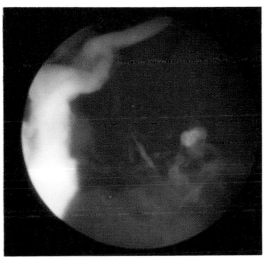

Arthroscopic view of blood in a joint—haemarthrosis.

Radiology—The usual special investigation is a plain radiograph. After physical examination the doctor must give the radiologist a history and differential diagnosis. Only in this way can a sensible report be provided (and the appropriate part be radiographed). For example, without examination of the injured wrist, radiographs of this joint rather than scaphoid views will be requested. Other investigations include ultrasonography and bone scanning, computed tomography, and magnetic resonance imaging, usually after referral to hospital.

Causes of haemarthrosis

- Torn anterior cruciate ligament (in 75%)
- Meniscus tear
- Chondral separation

Diagnosis—By now there should be a differential diagnosis and a favoured diagnosis. It is always slightly consoling that relatively few things can happen to joints and their surrounding structures.

Skin

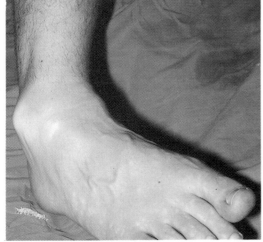

Ankle dislocation with skin at risk over the lateral malleolus.

In reviewing joints from the outside, start from the skin. Impacts over joints are common, and hard ground or artificial surfaces create appreciable skin lesions caused by shear forces. Such lesions may also be indicators of the underlying joint injury. In all cases they need to be cleaned and covered with a breathing adhesive drape that allows protected rapid healing.

Management of the acutely injured joint
Muscles

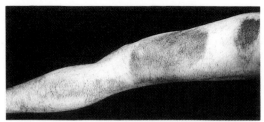

Intermuscular haematoma after a kick during a game of rugby.

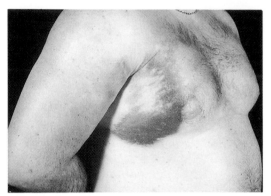

Intramuscular haematoma in a power lifter.

Muscle injuries

- Intermuscular haematomas
  Bruising (full length of limb), slight soreness, movement not (or only briefly) affected
- Intramuscular haematomas
  Profound long lasting stiffness
  Treatment regimen RICE (rest, ice, compression, and elevation)
- Strain
  To prevent the "second injury syndrome," ensure that lesion has healed before sport is started again

---

More deeply sited are contusions in and around muscles. These may produce very spectacular results indeed.

Intermuscular haematomas may produce bruising along the whole length of a limb simply because the blood tracks between the muscle belly and may reach the surface almost anywhere. Although joints may be sore, movement of them either remains full or rapidly returns to normal.

Intramuscular haematomas are bleeding contained within the muscle sheath, which can cause high pressures. This sort of injury therefore produces very profound stiffness that may also be slow to resolve. In all contusions of this nature the old RICE regimen (rest, ice, compression, and elevation (raising the affected part)) cannot be bettered. Rest must be tempered by the athlete's wish to return to sport and by the joint's need to return to movement. Rest the limb of the injured joint and encourage or allow the athlete to use the uninjured limbs and to maintain cardiovascular status. **Rest applies to the joint not the patient.** Ice (though its action is poorly understood) is traditionally used and seems to be effective. It has to be wrapped in a towel, not applied direct to the skin; an accessible source of the appropriate low temperature material is a bag of frozen peas straight from the freezer. Compression is commonly obtained using a crepe bandage but increasing use is being made of equipment capable of pulsing compression, such as the aircast system (Aircast, New Jersey, USA). The point of compression is to reduce the volume of the inflammatory fluid and permit the cells to restore normality without laying down fibrous tissue, which inevitably leads to stiffness. Raising injured joints is simply another way of achieving the same thing. A patient must be encouraged to move the joint in a small pain free range to maintain its mobility and promote healing.

Strains—Muscles can also be strained—that is, have a degree of longitudinal failure. Hamstring injury is typical; the muscle crosses two joints (the hip and knee), which commonly causes problems with coordination. Ligaments of major joints are relatively weak and depend on muscle control for their integrity. If major joints are heavily stressed before those muscles are in control the ligaments can be injured. This often happens after injury to the quadriceps if a player goes back too soon and then tears the ligaments in the knee—"second injury syndrome." Full muscle rehabilitation is essential before return to competition.

Ligaments

Sprains of ligaments

- *Grade I* (local tenderness, normal joint movement)
  Give NSAIDs, support sprain, encourage mobilisation
- *Grade II* (slightly abnormal joint movement)
  Give more protection, compression, and NSAIDs, raise affected limb; encourage middle range of movement (do not immobilise in plaster)
- *Grade III* (major abnormal joint movement)
  Refer to hospital, possibly examine under anaesthesia

Ligaments are also subject to sprains, which are usually graded into three degrees. Grade I sprains simply have some local tenderness over the ligament but there is no overt loss of integrity and the ligament is just sore. The treatment consists of explaining what is going on to the patient, non-steroidal anti-inflammatory drugs to help reduce the pain, and encouraging mobilisation (with an appropriate support such as a tubigrip).

Grade II sprains show slightly abnormal motion, which means that there is still overall integrity of the ligament but enough of it has been torn for it to stretch and it needs more protection. This is a perfect indication for the aircast system, ice, and non-steroidal drugs. This injury is perhaps seen most commonly around the ankle, where the anterior fasciculus of the lateral ligament often suffers a grade II injury. Early aggressive treatment in the middle range of movement with compression, elevation, and analgesia produces much better healing than plaster immobilisation, which frequently leads to failure of proprioception and a so called chronically unstable joint.

Grade III strains show major abnormal motion and must be referred to hospital for accurate assessment, possibly under anaesthesia.

Joints

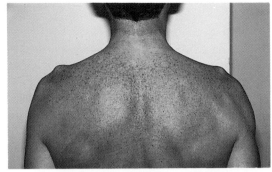

Subluxation of acromioclavicular joints (bilateral).

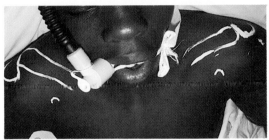

Marking to show dislocation of the acromioclavicular joint.

Reduction of dislocation or fracture

- Only if there are no complications (for example, neurological damage)
- Easier in recurrent dislocation
- Essential if a fracture causes pressure on skin
- Perform radiography afterwards to rule out fracture and (if there is no fracture, merely dislocation) to check whether reduction has been achieved
- Limit mobility and protect to help joint heal
- Exercise muscles across joint

Subluxations are incomplete dislocations where some degree of contact remains between the articular surfaces. A common example is a lesion of the acromioclavicular joint, in which some disruption of the capsule occurs but the main ligamentous structures remain intact. Few regular contact athletes have not had this injury. It is typified by a slight step deformity and does not require surgery. Subluxations should be distinguished from dislocations.

Dislocation implies complete loss of contact between joint surfaces and is a far more serious injury than subluxation. Continuing with the acromioclavicular analogy, the direction of displacement is not upwards but backwards and is best detected by accurate observation from above a seated patient. The most common dislocations are seen at the fingers, shoulder, patella, and elbow. Shoulder and elbow dislocations may be a little difficult to recognise immediately from observation, but those of the fingers and patella should be obvious. Careful palpation should show dislocations at other sites.

Depending on the doctor's skill and experience and how quickly after the injury the dislocation is seen, immediate reduction may be attempted. This may be easier in cases of recurrent dislocation (usually of the shoulder) but should be performed only in the absence of any complicating factors. These include any evidence of neurological damage; it is mandatory to test the circumflex nerve before reducing a dislocated shoulder. The neurovascular status must be checked and recorded after reduction. Rarely, a fracture dislocation of the ankle may press so hard on the skin that immediate reduction is essential to stop the skin dying. Once any reduction has been performed radiology is essential, even if done before reduction, to confirm the reduction and exclude any associated fractures.

Most dislocations can subsequently be safely mobilised within the middle range, protecting the torn structures from the extremes of movement while promoting better healing. Dislocated fingers are strapped to adjacent fingers or a double barrelled finger sized tubigrip is used, and early return to sport is allowed. A dislocated shoulder must be protected until adequate healing has taken place, and exercises to build up the muscles across the joint are essential.

Special circumstances

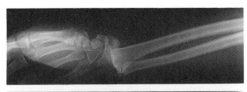

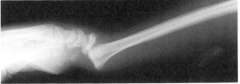

Complete separation of the distal radial epiphysis.

Immature skeletons—In childhood, ligaments are stronger than epiphyses. In the apparently unstable knee of a child the movement is often taking place at the distal femoral epiphysis. Stress radiographs must therefore be taken. The most common example of this injury is the "lateral ligament ankle sprain," where in fact the lateral fibular epiphysis has given way but has sprung back into position. This can be detected by careful palpation, and the tenderness will be found exactly over the epiphyseal line of the fibula rather than the ligaments themselves. This is perhaps one of the few indications for plaster immobilisation of "soft tissue" ankle injury.

Haemarthrosis of the knee—The importance of this injury is not well recognised. The history is usually of a non-contact twisting injury of the knee, often associated with an audible crack and followed quickly by swelling. With minor exceptions, radiographs of these joints show no abnormality. Until proved otherwise, rapid swelling indicates haemarthroses, three quarters of which are caused by torn anterior cruciate ligaments. The cause of bleeding in most other cases is a meniscus tear. As the meniscus has bled it has a blood supply and, if relocated and fixed (which is a quick and simple procedure viewed through an arthroscope), there is a good chance of it healing. A few have sustained a chondral separation. That can be relocated and fixed simply, which is essential to avoid exposed bone (as it can lead to osteoarthritis) in a young patient.

The photographs showing intermuscular and intramuscular haematomas appear (in black and white) in: Helal B, King J, Grange WJ, eds. *Sports injuries and their treatment.* London: Chapman and Hall, 1987. They are reproduced with the kind permission of the publishers.

MUSCULOSKELETAL INJURIES IN CHILD ATHLETES

Leslie Klenerman

Exercise is recommended for growing children. It stimulates the development of the musculoskeletal system. Physical activity regimens can enhance cardiovascular fitness in youngsters and offset the adverse effects of passive leisure activities like computer games. The general principles of an endurance training programme for adults can be applied to a programme for children. Nevertheless, training regimens should be conservative and emphasise the element of "play" and enjoyment. It is important that parents encourage physical activity in their children; furthermore, it is far more likely that the habit of regular exercise will persist if there is parental participation as well. If the parents exercise their children will follow their example.

The growing skeletons of children may be injured more easily than the mature skeletons of adults because the bones are more porous, and the long bones are further weakened by the epiphyseal plates at their proximal and distal ends. Children and young teenagers nevertheless have a lower injury rate from participation in sport than fully mature adolescents.

Injuries to epiphyses require precise reduction to prevent deformities. Crush injuries may result in uneven growth at the epiphyseal plate and produce angular deformities. If the whole epiphysis is damaged shortening of the limb may occur. All children who have had serious epiphyseal injuries require regular observation throughout the growth period.

Osteochondroses

Osteochondroses are a loose grouping of conditions affecting the growing epiphysis. They all show healing in radiographs. Common examples that occur in growing children at traction epiphyses are Osgood-Schlatter disease (at the tibial tuberosity), Sever's disease (at insertion of the Achilles tendon), Larsen-Johansson disease (at the lower pole of patella). Others that affect articular surfaces are Freiberg's disease (at the head of second or third metatarsal) and Panner's disease (at the capitellum). These disorders result because physical activity in vigorous growing children produces stresses at the junction of bone and ligament or on articular surfaces.

Osgood-Schlatter disease is caused by a traumatic avulsion of the patellar tendon from the tibial tuberosity and occurs commonly in children aged 11-13. There is pain and discomfort over the tibial tuberosity after exercise. Examination shows local tenderness and prominence of the tuberosity. The best treatment is to ignore the symptoms. Parents should be advised that symptoms usually last for 12-18 months. Rest will relieve the pain. If the children wish to be active they will aggravate their symptoms but come to no harm. Surgery is rarely required but may be necessary for excision of unfused ossicles deep in the ligamentum patellae. These cause pain on kneeling in adulthood.

Larsen-Johansson disease has a similar pattern of symptoms to Osgood-Schlatter disease but occurs at the lower pole of the patella owing to traction by the ligamentum patellae.

Sever's disease is similar to the two previous diseases but occurs in the heel just below the insertion of the Achilles tendon. There is traction on the growth centre by both the Achilles tendon and the plantar aponeurosis. There is no specific radiological appearance diagnostic of the disorder. The transverse and translucent zones seen on the radiograph are due to tension on the epiphysis.

Freiberg's disease entails collapse of the articular surface of the second or third metatarsal heads and is commonest in girls aged 12-15. There is pain on weight bearing, which results in reduced physical activity.

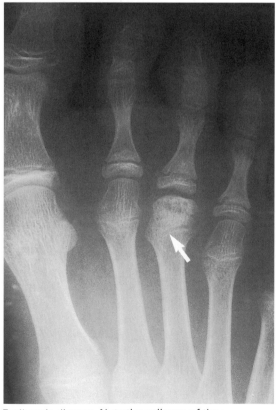

Freiberg's disease. Note the collapse of the metatarsal head and the sequestrum within the head.

Examination shows local tenderness, swelling, and pain on extension of the affected toe. Non-surgical measures, rest, and a metatarsal pad are often effective in relieving symptoms. Surgical treatment primarily entails removal of loose fragments of articular cartilage and should include resection of a small part of the dorsal aspect of the metatarsal head to allow free dorsiflexion at the metatarsophalangeal joint.

Fractures

Stress fracture diagnostic aids

- History of training
- Pain on ultrasound treatment
- Plain radiography
- Technetium bone scanning
- Computed tomography
- Scintigraphy

Stress fractures occur in children less often than in adolescents or adults. Common sites are the upper third of the tibia (51%), the lower third of the fibula (20%), and pars interarticularis of the lower lumbar vertebrae (15%). The primary training error that leads to stress fractures is doing too much too soon. Plain radiographs will provide the diagnosis in about 50% of cases. Scintigraphy misses few lesions and is invaluable when the diagnosis is in doubt. Stress fractures in the tibia have occasionally been mistaken for osteosarcomas. They occur most commonly in running and gymnastics.

Lesions of the pars interarticularis of the lower lumbar vertebrae occur in those subjected to hyperextension and high axial loading as occurs in gymnastics. In a study of 100 young female gymnasts the incidence of defects was 11%, which is about four times the incidence in the general female population (2·3%). Immobilisation in a plastic jacket will allow healing to occur if treatment is started early. Pars defects also occur often in young fast bowlers who are enthusiastic cricketers.

Another cause of back pain in adolescence is Scheurmann's disease. This is a disorder of growth associated with this age group, but does not occur as a result of excessive sporting activity. It is essentially the result of anterior disc herniation in the immature spine and may occur in both the dorsal and lumbar regions.

Shear stress and compressive loads have an important influence on physical growth. Obvious changes have been noted in the distal radial epiphyses of high level gymnasts. The extent of change is directly related to the intensity of training, and a reduction of workload will cause the changes to disappear.

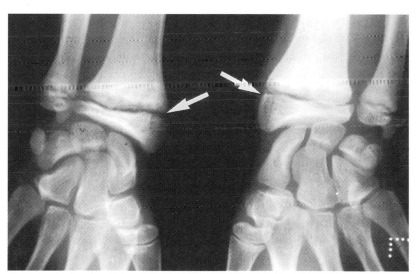
Changes in distal radial epiphyses of gymnast caused by shear stress and compressive loads.

Injuries of anatomical regions

Sports causing injuries of specific anatomical areas

Sport	Area at risk
Rugby	Neck (spinal cord)
Diving	Neck (spinal cord)
Mini-rugby	Hip (dislocation)
Swimming (butterfly stroke)	Shoulder
Throwing sports	Shoulder and elbow
Racket sports	Shoulder and elbow
General repetitive movements	Pelvis (overuse injury)

Head, neck, and spine

The incidence of major head or spinal cord injury in children under 15 is low. Damage is most likely to be in the neck. Rugby and diving are the commonest causes. Schoolboy rugby teams should be matched for size and weight rather than simply by age, as this policy reduces injuries. Scrum engagement still requires careful supervision, and crash tackling is illegal.

Shoulder girdle and elbow

Anterior dislocation of the shoulder is rare before the skeleton is mature. Occasionally, recurrent dislocation may occur and treatment is similar to that in adults by a Bankart or Putti-Platt repair. Impingement of the supraspinatus tendon beneath the coracoacromial arch is common in butterfly swimmers and in throwing and racket sports. The primary problem lies in the tendons of the rotator cuff and not in the coracoacromial arch. Impingement in young athletes is often secondary to shoulder instability.

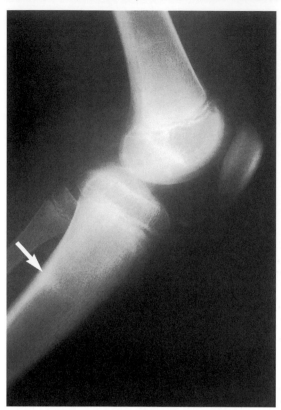

Stress fracture, upper third of tibia, lateral view.

Elbow

The main cause of elbow problems in athletes who throw objects are the valgus forces that are generated and which produce distraction on the medial side of the joint and compression on the lateral side. Osteochondritis dissecans may occur in the capitellum or radial head. Loose fragments require removal. Symptoms of pain in the elbow are common among young baseball players in North America. The throwing technique in cricket does not stress the elbow so much, so cricket does not impose the same high repetitive load on the elbow.

Wrist

Fractures and ligamentous injuries of the carpal bones are less common in children than in adults. The scaphoid is most commonly affected, most injuries occurring in children over 10.

Hip and pelvis

Overuse injuries from repetitive trauma occur around the pelvis. Pain may occur at any of the apophyses around the pelvis, on the iliac crest, the ischial tuberosity, or the anterior, superior, or inferior, iliac spines. Frank avulsion injuries sometimes occur at the surface of iliac spines; if wide separation results they may need open reduction and fixation. Sometimes late diagnosis of an avulsion of the ischial tuberosity is mistaken for an osteosarcoma. The lesser trochanter is sometimes affected and causes considerable pain and swelling. Treatment consists of rest, crutches, and physiotherapy.

Slips of the upper femoral epiphysis may present as either an acute or chronic condition. By definition only slips seen within three weeks of the onset of symptoms after trauma should be considered to be acute. This injury may occur in children aged 12-16 who have pre-existent mild chronic slips. An acute injury may precipitate displacement in a vulnerable capital epiphysis. Affected children are commonly either of the tall, thin, rapidly growing type ("greyhound type") or of the large and obese, hypogonadal type. The symptoms are of severe pain, limited movement, inability to bear weight, and an external rotation deformity of the leg. In chronic disease the child may complain of persistent knee pain and have no symptoms specifically related to the hip until a clinically noticeable slip has occurred. Early treatment is important before slips occur as it is difficult to fix the capital epiphysis by cannulated screws once moderate displacement has occurred.

Traumatic dislocation of the hip is not a common injury. Dislocations may result from athletic injury. Posterior dislocation of the hip has occurred in accidents during mini-rugby in which players kneeling on the ground have had someone fall on top of them. The incidence of complications of traumatic dislocation of the hip in children is lower than that in adults as the dislocation occurs with less force. Avascular necrosis may occur in about 10% of cases.

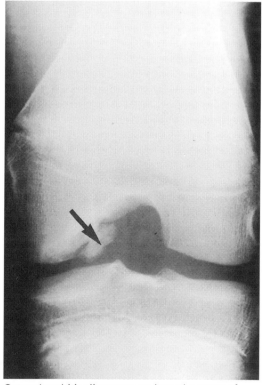

Osteochondritis dissecans on lateral a spect of medial femoral condyle.

Knee

Ligament and meniscal injury in children is rare but becomes more common as adolescence proceeds. Patellar instability and anterior knee pain are common. Osteochondritis dissecans is common in physically active adolescents. The lateral side of the medial femoral condyle is most commonly affected. Symptoms vary from discomfort on exercise to typical locking. In growing children the lesions may spontaneously reincorporate and disappear, whereas in older adolescents loose bodies may need to be removed.

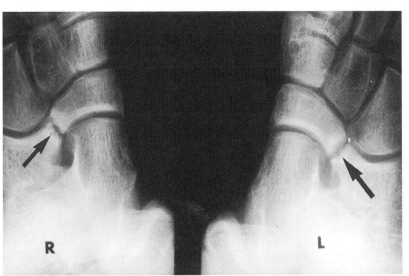

Bilateral calcaneonavicular bars not yet completely ossified, 45° oblique views of hindfeet.

Ankle and foot

So called sprains around the ankle are more likely to be epiphyseal injuries than to arise from ligaments. Tarsal coalitions—that is, calcaneonavicular or talocalcaneal bars—should always be considered in young athletes with persistent pain in the hindfoot. Examination will show rigidity of the subtalar joint. About 40% of tarsal coalitions present after injury. Calcaneonavicular bars are best seen in an oblique view (45°) of the hindfoot, but computed tomography is required to show talocalcaneal bars. Rest and reduction of activities may allow the symptoms to settle. If, however, pain and discomfort persist then excision of the bony bridge is indicated. Pain may arise from the sesamoids, which can be affected by traumatic fractures, stress fractures, and chondromalacia. Conservative measures to remove pressure from the painful area by means of a metatarsal pad are usually effective.

Conclusions

> **Preventing overuse injury in children**
> - Careful supervision by coaches and parents
> - Equipment checked regularly for fit and wear
> - Practice intensity and duration increased only gradually
> - Poor technique or posture recognised and corrected
> - Warm up and stretch exercises before and after sport

Children who actively participate in sport should not be treated as miniature adults: they need careful assessment in relation to the common problems that affect a growing skeleton. Overuse syndromes can be avoided by careful supervision from coaches and sensible parents. General practitioners should refer children who are keen athletes to orthopaedic surgeons as soon as possible to allow early treatment and to avoid a long interruption of sporting activities.

IMMEDIATE MANAGEMENT OF SEVERE INJURIES

James Graham

This chapter is a guide to the assessment and immediate care of the more common serious injuries from which participants may suffer at sporting events of all types. Head injuries have been discussed in a separate chapter.

Open (compound) fracture of a limb

The two elements in management of limb fractures are wound care and fracture care. An assessment should be made of the neurological and vascular state of the limb, particularly the vascular state as the degree of urgency in obtaining definitive treatment is greater if blood supply is disrupted.

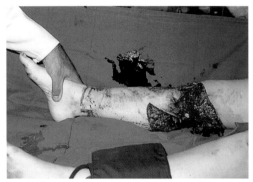
Extensive open fracture of the upper tibia.

Wound care

The main aim is reducing contamination by bacteria. Wherever possible foreign material should be removed from the wound provided that this does not cause any disruption of the tissues or undue pain. The wound must then be dressed to minimise further contamination. Ideally a sterile dressing containing antiseptic should be applied, but failing this any suitable clean material. Bleeding should be controlled by a dressing firmly bandaged in place and if possible by raising the limb after splinting. This measure can usually control most arterial bleeding, failing which pressure should be applied to the artery proximally and released every 10 minutes. A tourniquet should not be used.

Fracture care

Most fractures require splinting to control movement. The application of any splint is very difficult if not impossible if there is an angular deformity. Wherever possible any deformity should be gently and slowly corrected before the application of the splint. Splintage can be achieved by bandaging the limb to any firm straight object, such as a length of wood or a thickly folded newspaper, or by using an appropriate rigid or pneumatic splint. Arms can be splinted by the trunk and legs by the opposite leg.

Analgesia should be given by intravenous or intramuscular injection depending on the availability of an appropriately equipped doctor. Entonox is a suitable alternative.

Spinal injury

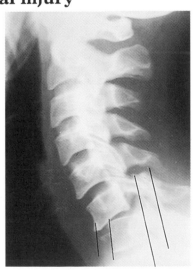
Dislocation of the cervical spine.

Most injuries of the cervical or thoracolumbar spine result from flexion and rotational forces. If the spine remains stable the cord is not at risk, but all spinal injuries must be regarded as being unstable until proved otherwise. If painless movement with normal sensation returns quickly after the injury, the spine is unlikely to be seriously affected. If pain and restricted movement persist in the absence of neurological symptoms or signs, the casualty should be referred to hospital for further assessment. The spine should be supported as follows: the cervical spine in a rigid collar and supported on either side by a sandbag or weight, or better still by a hand; the thoracolumbar spine on a rigid stretcher such as a scoop stretcher.

If the spinal cord is already injured (the patient has quadraplegia or paraplegia) the spine is unstable and care must be taken to avoid further injury. If there is a suspicion that there has been a transient or partial cord injury (indicated by paraesthesia, numbness, or weakness distal to the level of injury) the spine must be regarded as being unstable and be protected before transfer to hospital.

Cervical spine—Avoid flexing and rotating the neck. Keep the head supported by a hand on either side even when a rigid collar is used, as that only effectively controls flexion. Any movement of the casualty—for example, log rolling—must be done by several people maintaining the head, neck, and trunk in the same relationship at all times.

Thoracolumbar spine—Avoid flexing and rotating the spine. Any movement of the casualty, for example, rolling—should be achieved by several people log rolling the body keeping the shoulders and pelvis in the same plane throughout.

Any casualty with a spinal injury should be transported on a rigid stretcher. If the casualty is in any way trapped—for example, in a car—the above rules still apply. The spine must be maintained in the same relationship at all times, even if this means awaiting the arrival of cutting equipment to free the casualty. Special spinal splints are available for use in such instances.

Chest injury

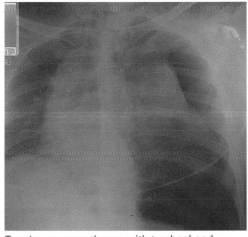

Tension pneumothorax with tracheal and mediastinal shift.

Serious chest injury results from either an object penetrating the thorax or a crushing force which results in multiple rib fractures with or without a flail segment. All may lead to loss of lung function with hypoxia either directly from the injury or indirectly from the development of pneumothorax or haemothorax. An acute deceleration injury may also result in disruption of the mediastinum. In all circumstances ensure that there is a patent airway with no obstruction.

Multiple rib fractures

The absence of paradoxical respiration must be confirmed. The casualty should be referred to hospital for further assessment, including radiography, to identify any developing complication.

Flail segment

If there is a segment of chest wall that shows paradoxical respiration the segment should be supported by a firm pad or hand to minimise the excursion of the segment. The risk of pneumothorax and haemothorax is high.

Penetrating injury

Pneumothorax is inevitable after a penetrating injury, either from air entering the wound or from an underlying lung puncture. A non-sucking wound should be dressed to effect a seal and a careful watch should be made for the development of a tension pneumothorax. A sucking wound should be dressed with a flap valve fashioned with a gauze swab over the wound and sealed on three sides. This minimises air entry from the outside yet allows release of any air from the pleural cavity, reducing the chance of a tension pneumothorax developing.

If a casualty with rib fractures, flail segment, or penetrating injury develops dyspnoea and increasing cyanosis that are associated with increased resonance of the chest on the affected side and a shift of the trachea to the opposite side, then a tension pneumothorax is probably developing. The tension urgently needs to be reduced, which can be achieved by inserting the widest bore needle available into the second intercostal space in the midclavicular line.

Mediastinal injury

If there has been an acute deceleration injury, such as occurs in a fall from a considerable height or a high impact collision, even if no chest wall fractures have occurred, it is still possible for the mediastinum to have been displaced, with injury to the aorta in particular. There may be no symptoms to indicate such a major mediastinal injury apart from some central chest pain. Such patients must be referred to hospital for further assessment. If bleeding has already occurred the patient will show signs of shock, and emergency transfer to hospital is mandatory.

Airway obstruction

The immediate care of airway obstruction can demand the highest standards of skill and experience to remove foreign bodies and achieve a patent airway by using the coma position or jaw thrust.

Causes of airway obstruction
- Facial fractures
- Foreign bodies
- Tracheal injury

Abdominal injury

Closed injuries from a heavy blow on the abdomen may cause rupture of a solid viscus (liver, spleen, or kidney) or tear the mesentery. Injury to the bowel is more likely from a penetrating wound, which may damage more than one viscus.

Closed injury

Serious injury is more likely from a blow to the upper abdomen, especially if pain and breathlessness (winding) do not settle quickly.

The casualty should be removed from the action and observed closely. If a closed injury is suspected the casualty should be admitted to hospital for observation because bleeding may occur later. Spreading abdominal tenderness should suggest the possibility of bleeding even in the absence of other general signs of blood loss. Rupture of the liver and spleen should also be suspected in association with fractures of the lower ribs on the right and left, respectively. Haematuria is an important finding and requires hospital assessment.

Penetrating injury

Any injury that results in penetration of the abdominal wall may have caused damage to any intra-abdominal structure leading to bleeding or peritoneal contamination, or both. The wound should be covered (preferably with an antiseptic dressing) and the casualty removed to hospital immediately. If bowel is protruding this should not be replaced but covered with a moist dressing.

> **Types of abdominal injury**
> - Closed
> - Penetrating

Pelvic injury

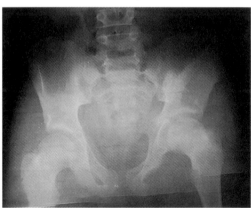

Unstable fracture of hemipelvis.

Serious pelvic injury results from either a fall from a height or a crushing force. They are identified by instability of the pelvic ring and are associated with extensive retroperitoneal bleeding and sometimes injury to the bladder and/or urethra.

It is not easy to splint pelvic injuries effectively, but if the pelvis is grossly unstable then a sand bag or similar item can be used to support each side behind the hip to minimise movement during transport to hospital.

Further reduction in movement can be achieved by bandaging the feet and legs together in a similar way to the splinting of tibial or femoral fractures.

Dislocations

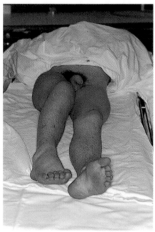

Attitude of leg with dislocation of hip.

Hip

Posterior dislocation results from violent force usually applied to the knee when the hip and knee are flexed—for example, dashboard injury in a head on collision. The leg assumes a position of flexion, adduction, and internal rotation at the hip, which usually cannot be altered. As a result splinting is difficult but should be attempted using the uninjured leg.

Knee

Dislocation of the knee is a rare injury, but is usually serious in that it is associated with a high incidence of injury to the popliteal artery. It results from a violent force applied to the knee, usually disrupting all the ligaments. If the dislocation is very unstable the deformity can be carefully corrected and the leg splinted as for a fracture. If the dislocation is "locked" the leg should simply be splinted for transport to hospital.

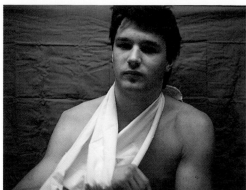

Dislocation of shoulder.

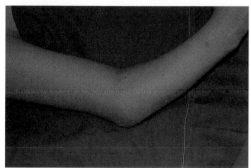

Dislocation of elbow.

Shoulder

The common anterior dislocation usually results from a fall on to the shoulder or from a violent twisting injury. It can be recognised by an angular appearance replacing the normal rounded shape. Immediate reduction should be attempted only by an expert and only if he or she is confident that there is no concomitant fracture. Otherwise the arm should be rested in a sling and this may be augmented by body binding, which splints the arm to the chest wall.

Elbow

The more common posterior dislocation usually results from a fall on to the outstretched hand, which pushes the forearm backwards on the upper arms. The elbow is held in the partly flexed position with the olecranon projecting posteriorly. Associated fractures are common, and reduction should therefore be deferred until radiographs have been taken. The arm should be splinted in the deformed position, or if possible rested in a sling, for transfer to hospital.

OVERUSE INJURY

Peter N Sperryn

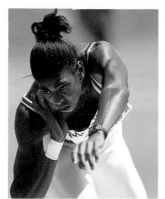

Overuse injury is common in shotputters.

The demands of training make overuse injury endemic in modern sport. High volumes of hard work underpin strength and stamina, while skills are honed through endless repetitious practice of event techniques.

Sports training and competition have intensified with the trend towards professionalism. For instance, many club level runners now cover some 50-110 kilometres a week, mostly on hard surfaces, instead of the previous generation's 30-40 kilometres. Field event athletes may train with weights of over 130 kg, and the scope for injury is obvious. Swimmers, often young adolescents, can train for several hours a day, and the physical, mechanical, and mental stresses are important factors in many youngsters' decisions to drop out of sports prematurely.

Overuse factors

Causes of overuse injury

- Load too great for conditions
- Technique or posture poor
- Equipment faulty or of poor quality
- Posture or anatomy inappropriate

Progressive resisted exercise—for training and rehabilitation

- Intensity of exercise increases gradually
- Loads increase slowly

(rather than starting exercise too intensively and increasing loads too fast)

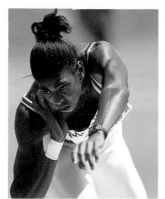

Cycling position—adjustable saddle and handlebars.

Load

An appropriate training load is one that the athlete is ready to manage on a given day but no ready definition exists of ideal or safe training loads. The concept of gradual and continuous training increments is central to the serious athlete's career development as well as safety. In today's sport, the winner is no longer the best athlete, but the one who succeeds in reaching the start—a statement well illustrated by the familiar pattern of outstanding athletes overtraining at the peak of their careers and breaking down in the run up to major competitions.

A training history is essential for the diagnosis and management of injury in athletes. Overuse injuries result from unaccustomed overload, such as going to training camps, working on new techniques, or being pushed by over ambitious coaches. More unexpectedly, simply returning to normal training after a rest long enough to "detrain" the tissues catches athletes unawares. The rule of "progressive resisted exercise" that governs medical rehabilitation also applies to training people with fit locomotor systems.

Technique

Technique is important to athletes. Axiomatically, the better the technique, the fewer the injuries (and the better the performance). Hence, if a doctor's role does not extend into coaching, he or she should at least recognise the need to refer an injured athlete to a competent event coach to clear up the current injury and to prevent its otherwise almost inevitable recurrence.

Posture

Posture is a key factor underlying injury related to movement, something long known in industrial medicine. There is often conflict between athletes' anatomy and the demands of their sports. In runners certain limb alignments and movement patterns predispose to injury. The importance of recognising such injuries is that their correction depends more on mechanical adjustment of running action than on medicine or physiotherapy.

Equipment

Equipment causes many overuse injuries, from arm strains due to faulty rackets to blisters from shoes, and equipment manufacturers are never far from the thoughts of sports physicians.

Combinations of factors

These factors—load, technique, posture, and equipment—may combine to cause pain and can be adjusted synergistically in treatment. For instance, knee pain in cyclists may be associated with cycling on a bicycle with a low saddle. Raising the saddle may relieve the symptoms by allowing the straighter leg action to balance better the strength of the quadriceps components and improve patellar tracking. Similar considerations apply to the backache that is common in cyclists, where judicious adjustments—up or down—of the saddle alter symptoms.

Preventing overuse injury

- Recognise and correct poor technique or posture
- Check fit and appropriateness of equipment
- Warm up and stretch before and after sport
- Gradually increase intensity and duration of practice

Types of overuse injury

Aids to diagnosing stress fracture

- History of training
- Pain on ultrasound therapy
- Plain *x* ray film
- Technetium bone scan
- Computed tomogram

Tissues prone to overuse injury

- Bones (stress fractures or metabolic overactivity)
- Joints (soreness, tenderness, restricted movement, effusions)
- Ligaments (overstrain)
- Muscles (stiffness, rhabdomyolysis) ⎫
- Tendons (overstrain, tenosynovitis) ⎭ (enthesiopathy at junctions with bones)

Bone

Bone suffers from overt stress fractures. Stress fractures are recognised by their history of localised "crescendo" type pain related to exercise. Early plain films are normal, although painful response to localised therapeutic ultrasound is a diagnostic pointer. It is essential to treat a stress fracture by rest from the causal activity. This must be continued after the usual early pain relief, which may give a falsely good picture and encourage resumption of training.

More worrying for the clinician is the range of stress or overload lesions falling short of plain *x* ray film diagnosis. This may show a more diffuse metabolic overactivity on technetium scanning in line with more widespread bone overload. The tibia may show this diffuse pattern in some runners with shin soreness. This must be separated from long flexor strain or compartment syndromes. The practical implication is that the "tibial overload syndrome" needs a very protracted spell of rest from loading. As this probably means a year off running, the athlete is entitled to scanning "proof" of diagnosis before such a long rest sentence.

Joints

Joints may become sore after exertion such as running on hard pitches in stiff boots. Clinically there may be joint tenderness and restricted movement. More serious lesions, such as infection or the adolescent hip disorders, must be excluded but a clear history of inappropriate overload is a basis for the diagnosis of overuse strain, though the pathological nature of the strain may be uncertain. Occasionally an effusion is seen after acute overtraining—for example, in the knee. This usually settles rapidly with rest. There is no indication for corticosteroid injection in these cases.

Ligaments

Ligaments are very often overstrained. Strains of the collateral ligaments of the knee and ankle provide much of the routine clinical load of "sports medicine." Such injuries may reflect faulty technique or posture that needs to be corrected for full recovery. For example, persistent running on the same side of a strongly cambered road may lead to chronic ankle ligament pain—on the "downside" lateral and "upside" medial collaterals. Appropriate advice often makes formal medical treatment unnecessary.

Enthesiopathy

Enthesiopathy describes strains of muscle, tendon, or ligament attachments to the periosteum. These may include wrist extensor strains in racket sports, tibialis anterior strain in young footballers, elbow epicondylitis in racket sports and golf, and some cases of runners' shin pain. Treatment is by correcting any sporting causes, rest, and physiotherapy, and these strains often respond well to local corticosteroid injection.

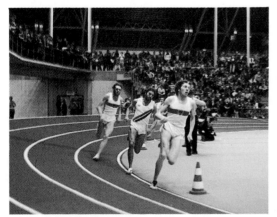

Indoor running—18 degree camber causes ankle strain.

Muscle

Muscle overuse starts with everybody's "stiffness" after unaccustomed exercise. More tennis elbows probably result from industrial work, gardening, or carpentry than from sport. Rhabdomyolysis may occur after severe exertion and, rarely, leads to serious illness including renal failure. It is also seen in marathon runners, some of whom have remarkable tolerance for, and recovery from, this form of severe tissue damage. Initial rest and lower exercise levels are the essential treatment for muscle soreness after exertion. The athlete should be advised on more gradual increments in future training. Despite extensive folklore, there is no established therapeutic benefit from heat, cold, or massage, and non-steroidal anti-inflammatory drugs have been shown to help only through their analgesic effects. Warming up and stretching before exercise help to raise muscle temperature and improve coordination. Stretching immediately after exertion is important in minimising subsequent stiffness.

Tendons

Tendons are often and painfully overstrained in sport. The typical acutely painful swelling of tenosynovitis follows acute overtraining and requires rest or immobilisation. The major tendons, the Achilles and patellar, have no formal synovial sheaths. They may become inflamed through simple overuse or because of friction—for example, from footwear rubbing on the Achilles. Chronic overuse injuries may be associated with focal necrotic lesions; chronic peritendinous fibrosis; and partial, sub-total, or complete ruptures. The importance of identifying any sporting cause is great as early diagnosis may prevent protracted disability.

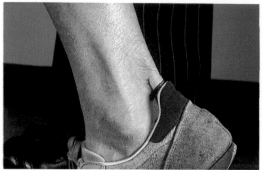

Achilles tendon pressure from shoe heel tab—note creasing.

Principles of management of overuse injuries

> **Treatment of overuse injury**
>
> - Rest affected part, but exercise remainder of the body
> - Non-steroidal anti-inflammatory drugs
> - Physiotherapy
> - Local corticosteroid injection (except intra-articularly)
> - Corrected or improved exercise technique

Firstly, correct the causes and apply compensatory "underloading." Rest need not necessarily be absolute. To athletes training intensively reduction from running, say, 150 kilometres a week on road to 50 kilometres on grass may relieve symptoms while allowing continued exercise. In other cases a lesion may be rested while a planned exercise programme can increase the load on all the other limbs. Athletes emerging from rehabilitation programmes often return quickly to, or exceed, their previous peak because they have switched from stereotyped and narrow overtraining regimens to more generally beneficial conditioning work, which provides a stronger basis for their special event endeavours.

Local physiotherapy methods are traditionally applied. Non-steroidal anti-inflammatory drugs may help in early and acute lesions—that is, when there is inflammation—rather than in long established chronic fibrosis. Local soft tissue corticosteroid injections are best reserved for injuries that have failed to respond adequately to the conservative methods of exercise correction, technique improvement, non-steroidal anti-inflammatory drugs, and physiotherapy. Intra-articular injection should never be undertaken lightly. Carefully supervised rehabilitation is essential after injection, as good initial response may be negated by precipitate overtraining while tissue is still healing. Accurate diagnosis and localisation are essential, and athletes should be told that, because corticosteroids weaken collagen, caution should apply especially towards premature resumption of heavy loading of the tendon at the lesion. For the same reason, direct injection into any tendon must be avoided.

The crux of the management of overuse injury is accurate recognition and correction of its sporting factors. Otherwise, resumption of the same training habits and sports techniques readily leads to demoralising recurrences. Time spent correcting faulty habits is well rewarded.

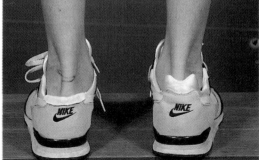

Achilles tendon protection—shoe surgery to relieve pressure from high heel tab.

The copyright for all photographs in this chapter except the first is with the author.

OSTEOPOROSIS AND EXERCISE

Roger L Wolman

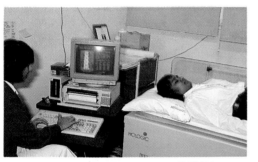

Exercise affects the skeleton in several ways. The direct effect of stress loading can be to increase bone mineral density, and this is now being considered as a strategy to prevent osteoporosis. Intensive aerobic exercise, however, can adversely affect bone density indirectly by its effect on the hypothalamic-pituitary-gonadal axis, which leads to a fall in blood oestrogen concentrations. This article discusses these effects.

For 100 years it has been known that bone tissue adapts to the stress loads to which it is exposed. During the past 20 years bone densitometry has made it possible to assess the effects of physical activity on the skeleton. Bone densitometry measures the calcium concentration within bone. Several methods are used to measure bone density: the most popular is dual energy *x* ray absorptiometry (DEXA) because it gives a highly reproducible result and exposes patients to only small amounts of radiation. It uses a pencil-thin beam of *x* rays that scan over a skeletal site to a detector on the opposite side of the patient. From this, an estimate is obtained of the calcium concentration of the scanned bone.

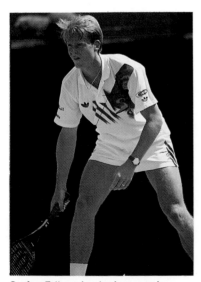

Dual energy *x* ray absorptiometry (DEXA) measurement of bone density.

Factors that increase bone density

Gravity (weight bearing)

Low levels of physical activity lead to a fall in bone density. Complete bed rest gives a negative calcium balance within a few days and a detectable reduction in bone density within a few weeks. This detrimental effect emphasises the importance of early mobilisation after acute illness or operation. The lack of gravity stimulation is thought to be responsible for the losses seen in the gravity free environment of astronauts. Though regular exercise is associated with an increase in bone density, this benefit is less pronounced if the exercise does not incorporate gravity stimulation. Thus swimming, being a weight supported activity, produces only a limited effect on the skeleton compared with some weight bearing activities.

Anatomical site of maximum stress

The skeletal response to exercise is greatest at the site of maximum stress. This effect is seen well in professional tennis players, whose playing arm can be up to 30% more dense than the non-playing arm. Large increases in bone density are seen at certain skeletal sites in athletes from other sports. For example, runners have increased bone density in the os calcaneous, femoral shaft, and spine compared with sedentary controls. Rowers, who perform intensive upper body exercise, display even more appreciable increases in spinal bone density.

Stefan Edberg's playing arm is considerably thicker than his non-playing arm.

Physical activity	Site of bone density increases
Running (jogging)	Os calcaneous, tibia, shaft of femur, spine
Tennis	Dominant arm, spine
Rowing	Spine
Volleyball	Spine, os calcaneous
Basketball	Spine, os calcaneous

Repetitive movements

Any exercise activity that produces repetitive stress loading to a part of the skeleton will tend to increase bone density at that site. The running action produces repetitive stress loading of the legs (800-2000 strides per mile (1·6 km) run—that is, 400-1000 repetitive loads on each leg), and this explains the impressive gains in leg bone density seen in long distance runners. Aerobic training, which usually entails continuous repetitive movements of two or more limbs, is associated with increases in bone density. Strength training, by stress loading a part of the body to build up muscle strength, also increases bone density.

Benefits of repetitive weight-bearing exercise

Intervention studies have shown that the prescription of these sorts of exercise programmes can lead to appreciable increases in bone density after several months of training. For older people exercise may reduce the risk of osteoporosis, even to people in their 80s. Exercise is not as effective as oestrogen replacement in postmenopausal women, but in older people exercise may also reduce the risk of osteoporotic fractures by improving muscle tone and balance, so reducing the risk of falls.

Adverse effects of intensive training

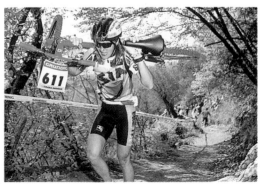

"Athletic amenorrhoea" in women

Aerobic exercise can affect the hypothalamic-pituitary-gonadal axis, thus leading to a reduction in oestrogen and progestogen release from the ovaries. The menstrual cycle may then become irregular or even cease. This "athletic amenorrhoea" was first described in the late '70s. Before then it was unusual for women to train sufficiently hard to develop amenorrhoea. With the increase in popularity of women's marathons, triathlons, and other endurance events, this disorder is becoming increasingly common.

Causes of hypothalamic-induced amenorrhoea

The cause of hypothalamic-induced amenorrhoea is uncertain. It is related to training intensity and to calorie restriction in the diet. A combination of these two factors leads to changes in body composition, in particular a reduction in body fat, and this seems to be a major influence in the development of amenorrhoea. Psychological stress may be a contributory factor, especially in competitive athletes. The incidence varies and is a reflection of the training requirements for each sport. Up to a half of the top class ballerinas, cyclists, runners, and rowers are amenorrhoeic.

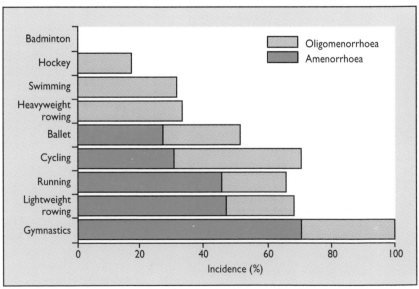

Proportions of women in various sports who have reduced or absent menstruation.

Up to half of the top class women ballerinas, cyclists, runners, and rowers have amenorrhoea and thus risk osteoporosis.

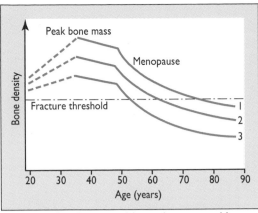

Bone density changes with age in women. Line 2=an average woman. Prolonged amenorrhoea in the 20s is likely to increase the risk of osteoporosis in later life (line 3). Conversely, intensive exercise in the 20s may reduce this risk (line 1).

Skeletal associations with low oestrogen concentration

- Reduced bone mineral density
- Stress fractures
- Delayed epiphyseal closure in adolescent athletes

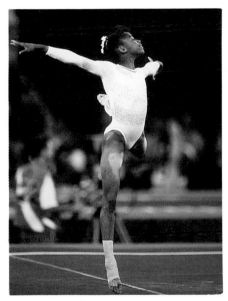

Some young women gymnasts and ballet dancers may have delayed menarche.

Effect of low blood oestrogen concentration on bone

Low oestrogen concentration has several effects on the skeleton, in particular a reduction in bone density despite high levels of exercise. The most important reduction occurs at sites where trabecular bone predominates (the spine and, to a lesser extent, the proximal femur and distal radius). With short episodes of amenorrhoea (up to six months) the fall in bone density is reversible, but if amenorrhoea is prolonged (two to three years) the loss may become irreversible. The risk of osteoporosis in later life is then likely to increase. In some athletes with prolonged amenorrhoea loss of bone density is pronounced and puts them at immediate risk of fracture. There have been some reports of insufficiency fractures occurring in athletes in their 20s.

Amenorrhoeic athletes have a higher incidence of stress fractures than their eumenorrhoeic counterparts. Although this may be due to low oestrogen, intensive training increases the risk of both stress fractures and amenorrhoea.

Effects of intensive aerobic training on men

There is some evidence to show that hypothalamic-pituitary-gonadal axis function in men who perform very intensive aerobic training is also disturbed, leading to a reduction in blood testosterone concentrations and sperm counts. The causes of this are probably similar to those in female athletes. Whether such male athletes are at increased risk of osteoporosis, however, has not been assessed.

Effects of intensive aerobic training on children

Intensive training in childhood may possibly delay the onset of puberty. Some gymnasts and ballet dancers may reach the age of 20 before menarche. This delay in menstrual function is associated with effects on skeletal maturation, with an increase in the risk of damage to the epiphysis.

Managing "athletic amenorrhoea"

Circumstances indicating referral of amenorrhoeic athletes to specialists

- Athletes with primary amenorrhoea (that is, aged 17 or older)
- Athletes in whom there is no clear cut association with training
- When amenorrhoea persists for more than six months

Assess whether exercise is the cause

The management of amenorrhoeic athletes can be difficult. In view of the effect on bone mineral density, this condition should not be regarded as benign. Any female athlete who has been amenorrhoeic for six months should be assessed medically. Initially it is important to assess the cause of the amenorrhoea. If her periods stopped when the athlete was increasing her training and started again when her training decreased (for example, during an injury) then the exercise was probably the cause.

Refer to gynaecologist, nutritionalist, or both

The relation with exercise intensity may not be clear cut, in which case a formal gynaecological opinion should be sought. Bone density measurement is important to calculate the degree of bone mineral loss. A nutritional assessment is also helpful as it will show whether the athlete's diet is deficient in calories or calcium, or both.

Treatment options

Dietary calcium deficiency should be corrected with either supplements or foods rich in calcium. Increasing the calorie intake may restore menstruation without an appreciable impairment in performance. The most effective way to treat this condition, however, is to get the athlete to reduce training intensity. Many will be unwilling to do this, in which case oestrogen replacement, in the form of either the oral contraceptive or hormone replacement therapy, should be considered. Some athletes are unable to tolerate hormone treatment, however, because of problems with fluid retention and the premenstrual syndrome. By this stage therapeutic options are limited, but at the very least athletes need to be warned about the potential long term risks associated with amenorrhoea.

Managing amenorrhoeic athletes

- Gynaecological assessment
- Nutritional assessment
- Reduction in training intensity
- Increase in calorie intake
- Consider oestrogen replacement (oral contraceptive or hormone replacement therapy)

Conclusion

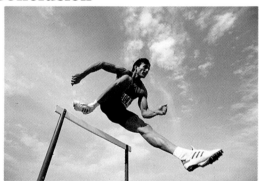

Exercise provides an additional method for preventing and treating osteoporosis. Athletes tend to have higher bone densities than the general population and can provide a model for assessing the effects of different exercise regimens on bone mineral density. Intensive aerobic training can, paradoxically, lead to a fall in bone density caused by low oestrogen. The exercise and oestrogen levels of a woman in her 20s and 30s may be very important in determining her eventual risk of developing osteoporosis.

The photograph of Stefan Edberg is reproduced with permission of Colorsport, that of the cyclist with permission of Professional Sport, that of the gymnast with permission of Allsport, and that of the hurdler with permission of Colorsport.

INFECTIONS

J C M Sharp

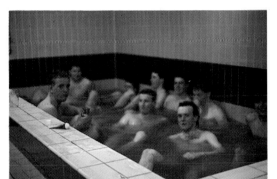

The widening range of sports and the ever increasing number of participants have meant that almost every type of infection may be acquired, directly or indirectly, in the pursuit of sport.

Though few if any of the more traditional sport associated infections, such as septic cuts, athletes foot, herpes gladiatorum, etc, have decreased in their occurrence, some new ones have recently emerged. Herpes has acquired an entirely new importance. There is also considerable concern regarding the possible risks of HIV and hepatitis B infection while participating in sport, particularly in combat and contact sports where blood may be spilt.

Increased attention has also been given to certain viral infections and their effect on athletic performance, and in particular to the debilitating effects of the Epstein-Barr virus (glandular fever) and coxsackievirus B infections, both of which have been associated with the chronic fatigue syndrome. In addition, premature return to active physical activity after influenza or similar feverish viral illnesses can have irreversible damaging effects on cardiac muscle.

In recent times sport has also become increasingly international as world travel has speeded up. In consequence more and more athletes (and officials) become exposed to a wider range of environmentally acquired infections such as "travellers' diarrhoea" in its various guises, viral haemorrhagic fever, malaria, etc.

During sporting activities

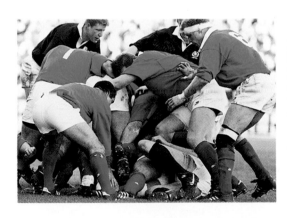

Infection may be acquired during sporting activities either direct by person to person spread (for example "scrumpox," hepatitis B, respiratory infections) or from contact with a contaminated field or pool (for example, sepsis, tetanus, leptospirosis, giardiasis)—with contact sports, water sports and field sports posing most risks. Indirect spread (for example, herpes, fungal infections) may also occur through sharing contaminated equipment, towels, or clothing.

Herpes gladiatorum ("scrumpox")

This condition caused by the herpes simplex virus is one of the most contagious of all infections, and outbreaks in sports clubs are common. Scrumpox is traditionally associated with rugby football; the presence of skin lesions combined with the abrasive effects of facial stubble while scrumming facilitate transmission of infection. Other causal combat sports include judo and wrestling. Infection may also be spread readily by sharing towels or equipment.

Treatment requires the use of acyclovir, a specific antiviral available as a cream or tablets. Prevention depends on maintaining high standards of personal hygiene and excluding infected players until successfully treated.

Scrumpox may also be due to bacteria (streptococci or staphylococci) or fungi (*Trichophyton* or *Microsporum*). Impetigenous forms of scrumpox are due to *Streptococcus pyogenes* or *Staphylococcus aureus*; erysipelas, the least common form, is potentially the most serious, with treatment requiring the use of antibiotics; tinea barbae spreads similarly to other forms of scrumpox, requiring treatment with fungicidal creams or tablets.

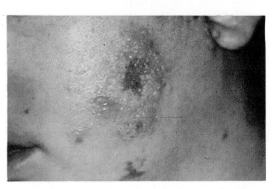

Herpes gladiatorum (scrumpox)—herpes simplex virus infection.

29

Infections

Specific antitetanus prophylaxis recommendations according to immunisation status and nature of wound

Immunisation status	Treatment if wound is:	
	"Clean"	Tetanus prone*
Basic 3 dose course or last booster dose within 10 years	Nil	Consider adsorbed vaccine if risk of infection is high
Basic 3 dose course or last booster dose 10 years or more ago	Booster dose of adsorbed vaccine	Booster dose of adsorbed vaccine + Human tetanus immunoglobulin
Not immunised or status uncertain	3 dose course of adsorbed vaccine	3 dose course of adsorbed vaccine + human tetanus immunoglobulin (given at a different site)

*(i) Any wound requiring surgical treatment that may be delayed for more than six hours.
(ii) Any wound with one or more of the following characteristics: an appreciable amount of devitalised tissue, a puncture type wound, contact with soil or manure likely to harbour spores, or evidence of sepsis.

Infections caught during sporting activity
- Scrumpox (herpes, impetigo)
- Wound infections (sepsis)
- Tetanus
- Waterborne (giardiasis, leptospirosis)
- Vectorborne (Lyme disease)
- ? Hepatitis B? HIV

Tetanus

Of all sport related infections, tetanus is potentially the most serious. Infection is caused by *Clostridium tetani*, the spores of which may frequently contaminate sports fields. Penetrating or "dirty" wounds facilitate bacterial growth and the production of neurotoxin. In Scotland within the past few years two rugby players and one soccer player developed tetanus from cuts acquired during play; only one of them, whose immunisation status was reportedly complete, survived. Treatment, other than for milder cases, requires intensive care providing sedation using curare-like drugs and life support facilities. Administration of antitoxin (specific antitetanus immunoglobulin) is necessary to neutralise any unbound toxin present, and penicillin is usually also required to eliminate any live bacteria capable of producing further toxin.

All wounds that are deep or dirty require early prophylactic treatment with thorough cleaning and debridement where necessary, complemented by penicillin and tetanus toxoid or antitoxin, depending on the immunisation status of the individual. Tetanus is readily preventable by active immunisation, with boosting doses recommended normally at 10 year intervals only. For rugby and soccer players and other athletes, however, who may be exposed frequently to potentially contaminated outdoor surfaces, additional boosters every 5-6 years or so should be considered while they are still participating actively. Too frequent booster doses may result in hypersensitivity developing and should not be pursued in people with a history of adverse local reactions.

Other wound infections

Any wound or abrasion may be infected by a range of bacteria (for example, *Staphylococcus, streptococcus, Pseudomonas*), which may be present in the playing arena or changing room, on clothing or equipment, on the skin, or in the respiratory tract of otherwise healthy carriers.

Water related infections

Water sports can pose infection hazards to various body sites or organs such as the eye (conjunctivitis, acanthamoebic keratitis), ear (otitis externa), skin (folliculitis), intestine (giardiasis, cryptosporidiosis), liver or kidneys (leptospirosis), or lungs (legionellosis), particularly in natural or unchlorinated waters.

Less common infections	Causal agent	Transmission	Incubation	Clinical presentation
Acanthamoebic keratitis	*Acanthamoeba polyphaga A castellanii*	Water (spas, hot tubs, etc)	Uncertain	Corneal lesion(s)
Cryptosporidiosis	*Cryptosporidium* sp	Untreated water (sewage effluents), person to person, farm animals, etc	1-12 days	Profuse watery diarrhoea, abdominal cramps
Giardiasis	*Giardia intestinalis*	Untreated waters (sewage effluents), person to person, wild animals, etc	5-25+ days	"Chronic" diarrhoea, loose greasy stools, cramps, malabsorption, etc
Legionellosis (Legionnaires' disease, Pontiac fever, etc)	*Legionella pneumophila L micdadei*, etc	Airborne droplets (air conditioning systems, showers, etc)	1-10 days	Headache, myalgia, fever, non-productive cough, atypical pneumonia (*L pneumophila* only)
Leptospirosis (Weil's disease, canicola fever, etc)	*Leptospira icterohaemorrhagiae L canicola*, etc	Via mucous membranes or skin abrasions from water contaminated with animal (rats, dogs, etc) urine	4-19 days	Sudden onset fever, headache, myalgia, conjunctival effusion, hepato-renal failure, meningitis, encephalitis
Lyme disease	*Borrelia burgdorferi*	Ticks (*Ixodes* spp)	3-32 days	Non-specific initially, followed by typical skin lesion(s) and neurological or cardiac symptoms, or both

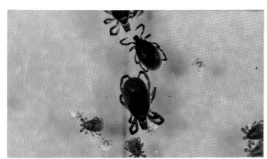

Ixodes ricinus (sheep ticks) are vectors for Lyme disease.

Vector borne infections

Bites of insects (such as ticks, mosquitos, etc) may cause a range of diseases in areas where Lyme disease, malaria, and other vector borne infections such as tick borne encephalitis, yellow fever, or Japanese encephalitis are prevalent. Cross country runners and orienteers may be particularly vulnerable. Lyme disease is caused by *Borrelia burgdorferi* acquired via bites from infected ticks of the *Ixodes* spp, occurs worldwide including Europe and the British Isles, and was originally identified in the United States where *I dammini* is the main vector. *I ricinus* ticks are widespread throughout the British Isles, particularly in woodland and bracken covered areas of the Scottish highlands, Wales, East Anglia, and the New Forest, where cases of Lyme disease have been reported.

In changing rooms

The shower and bathing areas of changing rooms, where athletes are crowded in a warm, moist atmosphere, are highly conducive to the transmission of a wide range of respiratory infections (influenza, sore throats) and fungal infections (tinea pedis, etc) or verrucas. Though most of such infections are merely nuisances, influenza not only incapacitates one person but can spread readily to fellow athletes, affecting performance and causing depletion of teams or cancellation of events. In addition, in a mistaken attempt to compete or to "not let the side down," affected athletes may try to "run off" their flu, the effects of which may be counterproductive to the team and potentially dangerous to the individual.

The damaging effects of certain viral infections on cardiac muscle is well recognised. Influenza type A virus has been isolated from the myocardium of people who died after flu-like illnesses, and its effects on the metabolism of heart muscle has been shown experimentally in mice. Myocarditis caused by *Chlamydia pneumoniae* (TWAR (Taiwan acute respiratory disease) agent) was shown to have caused sudden death in an elite Swedish orienteer. Other microorganisms, particularly enteroviruses (coxsackieviruses A and B, echovirus), parainfluenza virus, cytomegalovirus, and *Mycoplasma pneumoniae* and bacteria such as *Streptococcus* group A and *B burgdorferi*, are also known for their myocardiopathic effects.

The longer term debilitating effects of some viral infections such as influenza, measles, chickenpox, infectious mononucleosis, and the coxsackievirus group of enteroviruses have become recognised as being associated with the chronic fatigue syndrome. Particular attention has been given to the Epstein-Barr virus and the coxsackievirus group, both of which are known to affect muscle and nerve tissue.

Infections caught in changing rooms

- Athletes foot (tinea pedis)
- Verrucas
- Influenza, sore throats
- Glandular fever, which may lead to:
  Myocarditis
  Chronic fatigue syndrome

Viruses that may cause chronic fatigue syndrome

- Enteroviruses (especially coxsackie group B)
- Epstein-Barr virus
- Others—varicella, measles virus
- ? Yet to be identified

During travel abroad

The expansion of air travel has made accessible more countries worldwide in which a myriad of infections no longer present in Europe are still prevalent. Only smallpox has been eradicated on a global basis. The most common problems likely to be encountered outside western Europe, North America, and Australasia are gastrointestinal infections ("travellers' diarrhoea," salmonellosis, dysentery), viral hepatitis A, etc. In addition, the potential of contracting poliomyelitis in developing countries should not be underestimated.

Despite intensive efforts towards eradication, malaria has been increasing in recent years in Africa, Asia, and South and Central America in parallel with resistance of the mosquito vector to insecticides. In areas of South East Asia, South America, and Africa, strains of *Plasmodium falciparum* have developed resistance to chloroquine and other drugs, presenting further problems in prophylaxis and treatment.

Infections contracted abroad

- Brucellosis (goats' milk cheeses in Mediterranean countries)
- Bubonic plague (central and South East Asia, southern Africa, southern America, western states of the United States)
- Cholera
- Hepatitis B, HIV (worldwide)
- Malaria
- Poliomyelitis
- Rabies (worldwide)
- "Travellers' diarrhoea"
- Tuberculosis (worldwide)
- Typhoid
- Typhus (Far East and northern Australia)
- Viral haemorrhagic fevers (including Lassa fever) (West Africa)
- Yellow fever

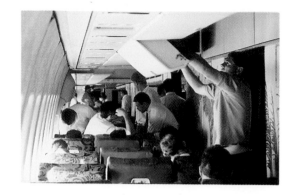

Respiratory illnesses are also particularly common among air travellers (who are exposed to airborne infection in crowded aircraft, airport terminal buildings, or hotels) and are compounded by the dehydrating effects of low humidity in aircraft.

During leisure time activities

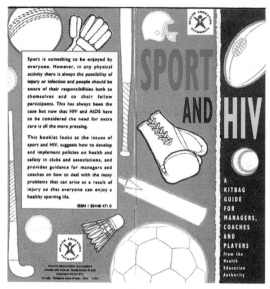

Leaflet produced by Health Education Authority.

Relaxing in or around a swimming pool or whirlpool may result in exposure to a range of environmentally acquired diseases, particularly respiratory or fungal infections. Other leisure time activities may result in a sexually transmitted disease. Of these both hepatitis B and HIV infection have the potential of being acquired through any one of sport related situations, although the relative risks vary from very low while actively participating in sport to increasingly likely as a consequence of some leisure time activities.

Hepatitis B virus (HBV)

Infection is most usually acquired through contact with infected blood (via shared needles, needlestick injuries, etc) or by sexual spread from a carrier of the disease. Chronic carriers, detectable by the presence of hepatitis B surface antigen in their blood, rarely have a recognisable illness yet they can remain infectious for many years. The main emphasis in sport is on improving overall hygiene standards rather than imposing undue restrictions on known HBV carriers. Such people need not categorically be excluded from participating in sport. Injuries, cuts, or grazes that bleed are nevertheless potential sources of infection and should be cleaned and securely covered immediately.

The risk of acquiring hepatitis B during sporting activities is small, but infection associated with thorn-pricks during orienteering events and among barefoot runners has been reported.

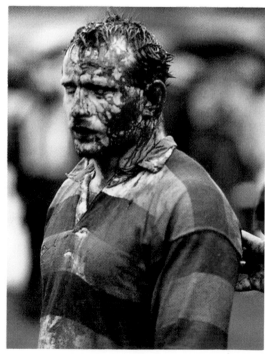

Bleeding players should not play on.

HIV infection

Although considerably less readily transmissible, the modes of acquiring HIV are virtually identical to those of HBV. In the United States, HIV antibody testing is mandatory in some states for all boxers, while in other states ringside "seconds" are required to wear plastic gloves.

Several instances of direct bloodborne person to person spread of HIV infection within families have been reported in the United States. While the risk of acquiring HIV infection is low, seroconversion was reported from Italy in 1990 in a previously healthy soccer player with no admitted risk factors, whose head had collided with an opponent's (an injecting drug user known to be HIV positive), resulting in both players bleeding copiously.

With this one apparent exception, there remains to date no evidence worldwide of the transmission of either HIV or HBV infection while participating in sport. Cuts or abrasions during sporting activity clearly require immediate attention and bleeding to be controlled before players return to the field of play. In rugby union, the laws of the game require that "a player who has an open or bleeding wound must leave the field of play until such time as the bleeding is controlled and the wound covered or dressed," with a temporary replacement being permitted. More recently, the International Rugby Football Board has prepared guidelines specific to bloodborne infections and contact sports.

Preventive measures

A wide range of prophylactic measures (vaccines, toxoids, immunoglobulin, antimalarial drugs, etc) are available against many infections. Most athletes nowadays should have had a basic course of tetanus toxoid in childhood, with subsequent booster doses to maintain effective immunity. Influenza vaccines should also be considered, although immunity is poorly maintained and repeat doses are required frequently.

Specific advice on prophylaxis, in particular against malaria, is always necessary for overseas travel outside western Europe, North America, and Australasia. Vaccines are available against typhoid, hepatitis A, and hepatitis B infections and should be considered for athletes competing in areas of the world (South America, Africa, the Far East, etc) where disease is endemic. Cholera vaccine, however, is now regarded as being ineffective in providing adequate protection. Vaccines are also available for some vector borne infections such as yellow fever (tropical Africa and South America), Japanese encephalitis (Far East), and tick borne encephalitis (central Europe, some areas of Scandinavia) but may not always be necessary for short stay visitors or at certain altitudes or seasons of the year. There is no vaccine for Lyme disease, and the value of protective clothing and repellent creams in preventing insect bites generally cannot be overstated.

Preventing infection in sport depends on many factors, among which maintaining good standards of personal and environmental hygiene are of paramount importance. Showering is always preferable to communal baths. Buckets and sponges are no longer acceptable and should be replaced by disposable wipes.

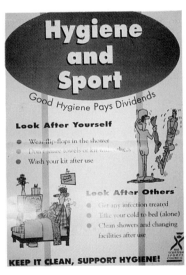

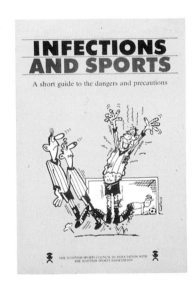

In recent years excellent guidelines on hygiene in sport for athletes have been produced by various organisations in the United Kingdom, including the Sports Council of Wales, the Scottish Sports Council, and the Health Education Authority. The Scottish Sports Council has also prepared a more comprehensive review entitled *Infections and Sports*.

Leaflet produced by Scottish Sports Council.

Recommended further reading

G R McLatchie, ed. *Essentials of Sports Medicine.* 2nd ed. Edinburgh: Churchill Livingstone, 1993:112-25.
E Walker, G Williams, F Raeside, eds. *ABC of Healthy Travel.* 4th ed. London: BMJ Publishing Group, 1993.

The photograph of a scrum is reproduced with permission of the *Glasgow Herald/Evening Times*, that of ticks with permission of Professor N R Grist, Glasgow, and that of an injured player with permission of Colorsport. The table on prophylaxis against tetanus was adapted from *Immunisation Against Infectious Diseases.* London: HMSO, 1992.

PULMONARY LIMITATIONS TO PERFORMANCE

Mark Harries

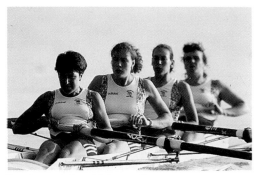

Rowing requires high ventilatory capacity.

Assuming lung function to be normal, there is said to be no pulmonary limitation to aerobic performance. Justification for this statement rests with the fact that, while exercising at the maximum aerobic capacity (that is, when the rate of oxygen consumption cannot be further increased (VO_2max)), it is possible to increase ventilation still more by voluntary effort. The main limiting factor is held to be a failure to match the rate at which muscle can consume oxygen with the rate at which oxygenated blood can be delivered; in other words, the cardiac output.

The lungs may be regarded as the carburetter of the engine, thus only when they are diseased—such as in chronic bronchitis or emphysema—does ventilatory capacity become reduced to the point where it limits exercise tolerance. Chronic bronchitis causes obstruction to air flow which, coupled with a reduction in vital capacity, results in a low ventilatory capacity or minute volume. Emphysema imposes an additional burden because not only is minute volume reduced but so also is oxygen transfer because of a loss of alveoli.

Importance of high ventilatory capacity

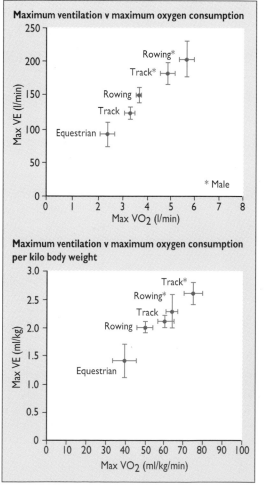

High ventilatory capacity is essential for sports such as rowing, cycling, and middle and long distance running. When exercised to maximum most elite athletes in their mid-20s reach a respiratory rate of around 55 breaths a minute with a heart rate of close to 200, regardless of their size. In absolute terms the highest minute ventilation is usually achieved by the biggest athletes, as breath volume is directly related to size. Indeed the highest so far measured at the British Olympic Medical Centre is 245 l/min clocked up by a male heavyweight rower. The same is also true of peak oxygen consumption, with the biggest athletes recording up to 8 litres of oxygen consumed a minute and an average around 5·26 l/min.

A more objective measure of aerobic performance is reached by removing the variability introduced by size by dividing by body weight. The minute ventilation of elite male track athletes is then about 2·7 l/kg/min with a maximum oxygen consumption of around 79 ml/kg/min. The relation between maximum aerobic capacity and minute ventilation is roughly linear. In other words people with the highest aerobic capacity tend also to achieve the highest minute ventilation.

Minute ventilation (VE) at maximum oxygen consumption VO_2MAX) in 120 Olympic class athletes. Those with the highest VE (male rowers) also have the highest (VO_2MAX) because they are the biggest. When the size factor is removed male track athletes score highest.

Airflow obstruction limiting performance

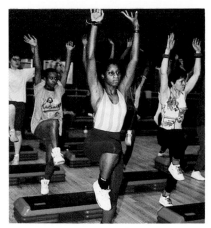

Exercise can induce asthma.

Minute ventilation is limited in respiratory diseases characterised by obstruction to air flow. Chronic obstructive airways disease may cause such severe ventilatory impairment that exercise tolerance is judged only by the distance covered when walking briskly on level ground for 10 or 12 minutes.

For athletes, asthma causing airflow obstruction holds a position of great importance because it is a common complaint. Of all those attending the British Olympic Medical Centre last year with underperformance not attributable to injury, around 20% blamed their poor performance on respiratory symptoms. But asthma is important for other reasons: obstruction to airflow can be brought on by exercise itself, and the reduced ventilatory capacity can readily be improved with treatment, thereby transforming performance.

Diagnosis of asthma

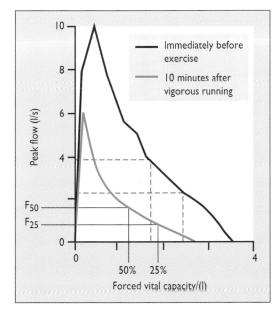

A history of cough or wheeze after exercise and particularly of sleep disturbance due to tightness in the chest should arouse suspicion. Diagnostic proof rests with showing an obstruction to air flow that is variable, so a minimum of two estimations of peak flow or FEV_1 (forced expiratory volume in one second) taken at different times of the day is needed. For normal subjects the variation in peak flow is seldom more than 8%, with the lowest measurement recorded usually first thing in the morning. Differences of more than 20% in values obtained at any time during the day is strongly suggestive of asthma.

Flow loop spirometry is performed with the subject breathing out forcibly from full inspiration to full expiration, giving forced vital capacity (FVC).

Exercise induced asthma in a track athlete. The flow loops measured before and 10 minutes after vigorous running show the typical changes with reductions of more than 15% in both peak expiratory flow and forced vital capacity. The peaking and sagging of the downward limb are important diagnostic signs. The sagging results in a bigger percentage fall in flow when both 50% and 25% of forced vital capacity remains to be expired (F_{50} and F_{25} respectively) than in FEV_1. In this instance FEV_1 fell 40% but F_{50} fell by 60% and F_{25} by 65%.

Exercise testing for asthma

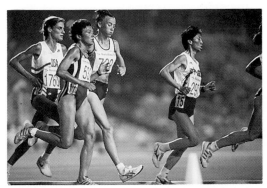

Running in the open air can cause bronchial constriction.

There is no agreed standard test protocol for inducing asthma with exercise, but certain ingredients are important. Running in the open air is a more potent stimulus to bronchial constriction than exercising on a bicycle or treadmill ergometer. The reasons for this are complex and are related in part to climatic conditions. Cold dry air causes more bronchial constriction than warm moist air. The exercise must be vigorous, sufficient to raise the heart rate to around 80% of the maximum that can be achieved (220 minus age in years).

The duration of the test is also important. It should last at least three minutes but not much longer than five. Either peak flow or FEV_1 can be measured with readings taken immediately before and at five and 10 minutes after the run. Normal subjects may show a short lived bronchial dilatation on stopping, but a fall of 15% or more from pre-test values is a positive result.

Improving performance with treatment

International Olympic Committee's Medical Commission's rules on antiasthma drugs

Drug class	Banned	Permitted (by inhalation only)
Corticosteroids	All oral, intramuscular (depot), or intravenous preparations	Budesonide (Pulmicort) Beclomethasone (Becotide)
Selective β adrenoceptor stimulants	All oral, depot, or intravenous preparations and fenoterol (Berotec) inhalation	Salbutamol (Ventolin) Terbutaline (Bricanyl)
Non-selective adrenoceptor stimulants	Ephedrine Isoprenaline (Medihaler)	
Antimuscarinic bronchodilators	None	Ipratropium (Atrovent) Oxitropium (Oxivent)
Cromoglycate preparations	Cromoglycate with isoprenaline (Intal compound)	Cromoglycate (Intal) Nedocromil (Tilade)
Theophylline	None	

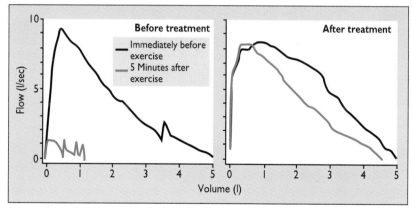

Severe bronchoconstriction induced by exercise. Both peak flow and forced vital capacity are greatly reduced. (Oscillations in the expiratory flow loop are the result of coughing.) After prednisolone 30 mg a day for two weeks the bronchoconstriction had been almost eliminated.

The photograph of the women's coxless four in the Olympic regatta at Bayolas, Spain, in 1992 was taken by Peter Spurrier, Sports Photography; that of Liz McColgan in the 10 000 m heats at the Barcelona Olympics in 1992 by Professional Sport; and that of a step aerobics class by Richard J Sowersby.

Effective treatment of airflow obstruction undoubtedly improves performance. However, some athletes have unrealistic expectations. Paradoxically the greatest problems arise when an individual has been given treatment for which there is no indication. The problem then becomes one of withdrawing medication. Selecting a drug regimen that will not violate the doping regulations of the International Olympic Committee (IOC) is crucial. As a rule of thumb, all systematically acting antiasthma drugs are banned whether taken by mouth or parenteral injection, the only exception being aminophylline.

The mainstay of treatment in asthma, of which exercise induced bronchial narrowing is a symptom, is corticosteroids by inhalation. Both budesonide and beclomethasone are permitted, and the dose should not exceed 1600 μg a day. Powdered preparations are longer acting than metered dose inhalers and effective when taken morning and evening. Bronchodilators form an adjunct to inhaled steroids and are best taken around 10 minutes before competition. Selective β agonists such as salbutamol and terbutaline are permitted, but fenoterol is banned. Bronchodilators with stimulant properties such as adrenaline and isoprenaline are also banned.

Sodium cromoglycate inhibits exercise asthma if taken about 10 minutes before competition and is especially effective in children. The combination of cromoglycate with isoprenaline is a banned substance and must not be used.

Caveat

At present any athlete is able to obtain antiasthma medication and is allowed to inhale any amount that he or she pleases. There is no obligation to provide medical evidence of respiratory disease. As a result, some athletes are taking medication only because they have been told by fellow competitors that it improves performance. I have seen one who was in the habit of taking 20 puffs from a salbutamol inhaler before each race. The IOC Medical Commission has yet to rule on this issue, and until it does the situation will remain unsatisfactory.

THE OVERTRAINING SYNDROME

Richard Budgett

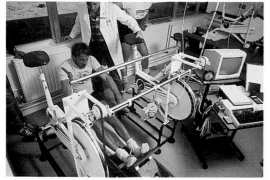

Wingate test using rowing machine. (Steve Redgrave, triple Olympic winner.)

Athletes may experience chronic fatigue for many reasons, but it often results from the stress of training and competition—when it is called the overtraining syndrome. The primary complaint is of reduced performance, which is objective and can be measured. Many athletes train at an elite level even to compete domestically, so fatigue due to the stress of training is not confined to Olympic athletes; 10% of college swimmers in the United States are described as "burning out" each year.

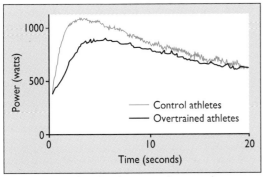

Wingate test showing lower peak power in overtrained athletes.

The cause of the overtraining syndrome is not known and there is no diagnostic or warning test. Intensive interval work (high intensity exercise with little rest) is most likely to precipitate the syndrome, so it is extremely rare in sprinters because they train with large amounts of rest. Sprinters may, however, suffer from postviral and other forms of chronic fatigue.

Definitions

Overtraining—hard training without adequate rest (pathological)

Over-reaching—hard training with adequate rest (normal)

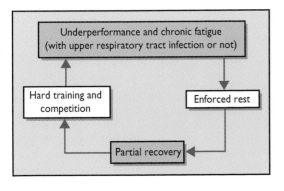

Overtraining
Overtraining is the process of excessive training that leads to the overtraining syndrome, which can be defined as a state of prolonged fatigue and underperformance caused by hard training and competition. There should be an objective measure of the loss of form, which will have lasted at least two weeks despite adequate rest and will have no identifiable medical cause. Symptoms of a minor infection, typically an upper respiratory tract infection, may recur each time the athlete returns to training after inadequate rest.

Over-reaching
Over-reaching is the process of hard training that enables athletes to reach their full potential. It is part of a planned programme to stimulate adaptation and, when combined with periods of rest, permits the normal physiological response of full supercompensation. This contrasts with the pathological response to training in the overtraining syndrome.

Presentation

Precipitating factors of the overtraining syndrome

- Training
  —Intensive interval training
  —Sudden increases
  —Large volumes of monotonous training
- Stress of competition and selection
- Physical stresses
  —Glycogen depletion
  —Dehydration
  —Other illness or injury
  —Psychological stress of life events (for example, moving house, exams, relationship problems)

Symptoms of overtraining

- Underperformance
- Depression (loss of purpose, competitive drive, and libido)
- Loss of appetite, and weight
- Increased anxiety and irritability
- Fatigue
- Sleep disturbance (in over 90% of cases)—difficulty getting to sleep, waking in the night, nightmares, and waking unrefreshed
- Frequent minor infections, particularly of the upper respiratory tract
- Raised resting pulse rate
- Excessive sweating

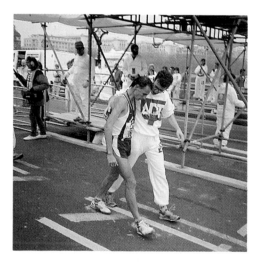

Signs of over-reaching (which is normal if athletes recover quickly)

- High serum creatine kinase concentration
- Low ratio of serum testosterone to cortisol concentrations
- Falls in muscle glycogen concentration
- Raised resting heart rate
- Mood deterioration

Symptoms

Athletes present with fatigue, heavy muscles, underperformance, and depression. Direct questioning reveals poor sleep in over 90% with difficulty getting to sleep, nightmares, waking in the night, and waking unrefreshed, which may be important in the pathogenesis. Other symptoms are loss of purpose, energy, competitive drive, and libido; emotional lability; increased anxiety and irritability; loss of appetite with weight loss; excessive sweating; and a raised resting pulse rate. Some athletes keep catching minor infections every time they build up their training.

Training stresses

The history usually involves an increase or change in training.

Intensive interval work—Many athletes break down when they switch from low intensity winter training to high intensity summer training with intensive interval work. The stress of competition and selection pressures may also contribute. The athletes can usually keep up at the beginning of a race but describe an inability to lift the pace or sprint for the line.

Fast athletes—Some athletes are going faster than ever before but think that training even harder is the only way to achieve even greater success, so they cut recovery time to permit more training and competition. One swimmer broke the British record and then decided to cut his rest day to train seven days a week instead of six. He broke down after several months and took many weeks to recover. Another swimmer increased his training to eight hours a day; for four months his performance improved, but then he started to fail to recover from training and took months to recover form.

Slow athletes—Others are trying to keep up with peers who are faster, so the stress of training is greater and they become fatigued. It is difficult for them to accept the diagnosis because they are training less than other competitors, but it is their individual response to training that matters.

Sudden increase—Some suddenly increase their training in order to catch up after a break due to illness or injury when it would be sensible to increase training gradually. They get more desperate and train harder as they fall further behind.

No periodisation of training—Occasionally training may be heavy, monotonous, and without periodisation (cyclical variation of training).

Other stresses

Stresses such as exams and other life events, glycogen depletion, and dehydration will reduce the ability to recover from, or respond to, heavy training. However, it is rare for athletes to break down after less than two weeks of hard training (as in a typical training camp) provided that they then rest and allow themselves to recover afterwards.

Signs

These are inconsistent and generally unhelpful in making the diagnosis. They include increased postural drop in blood pressure and postural rise in heart rate, slow return of the pulse to normal after exercise, decreased lactic acid levels during exercise, reduced maximum oxygen uptake and maximal power output, and increased submaximal oxygen consumption and pulse rate.

Investigation

Exclusion of other causes of chronic fatigue

- History—inquire about infection, wheeze, eating disorders, chest pain, and shortness of breath on exercise
- Examination—to exclude a medical cause
- Investigation—depends on clinical possibilities. May include lung function and laboratory tests

---

Overtraining may cause immunosuppression by:

- Raised serum cortisol concentrations
- Low serum glutamine concentrations
- Low salivary IgA concentrations

Laboratory tests rarely help in the diagnosis of chronic fatigue

---

It is often difficult to persuade athletes and coaches that overtraining has caused underperformance. Investigations are needed to exclude other causes of chronic fatigue and to convince an athlete that there is no undiagnosed illness. The range of these tests depends on a sensible approach to clinical possibilities. Serious disease such as viral myocarditis and arrhythmia is rare but must be excluded if suspected. Prolonged glycogen depletion, as in anorexia nervosa, may cause chronic fatigue in its own right. A history of recurrent upper respiratory tract infections may represent allergic rhinitis or exercise induced asthma, in which case lung function tests are needed.

Laboratory tests

Laboratory tests are occasionally helpful but their use in diagnosing and monitoring chronic fatigue in athletes has been overrated.

Haemoglobin concentrations and packed cell volume decrease as a normal response to heavy training. An athlete's reported anaemia is often physiological, due to haemodilution, and does not affect performance. Increasing the haemoglobin by altitude training or blood doping (cheating), however, does seem to improve performance.

Ferritin—It is controversial whether low serum ferritin concentrations (which reflect low iron stores) can cause fatigue in the absence of anaemia. If the ferritin concentration is very low, however, treating an athlete with iron by mouth is reasonable.

Creatine kinase—There is a wide individual variation (50-fold) in the response to hard exercise. Serum concentrations above 2000 mmol/l have been seen in normal marathon runners and do not indicate who will break down with chronic fatigue.

Viruses—Viral titres must be shown to rise, and the history is normally suggestive of a post-viral illness. The Paul-Bunnell test is diagnostic and there may be high serum levels of enteroviral particles.

Trace elements and vitamins—There is no proved link of vitamin or trace elements to the overtraining syndrome, and the widespread use of supplements by athletes does not seem to offer any protection from chronic fatigue.

Prevention and early detection

Profile of mood state (POMS) graph showing normal iceberg profile and abnormal inverted iceberg profile in overtrained athletes.

Early detection of overtraining syndrome is difficult

Monitor: Performance

Mood state

Resting heart rate

Athletes can tolerate different levels of training and competition stress; overtraining for one may be insufficient training for another. Each athlete's tolerance level will also change through the season so training must be individualised and varied and should be reduced at times of other stresses such as exams. Unfortunately athletes are exhausted most of the time unless they are tapering for a competition, so it is difficult for them to differentiate overtraining from over-reaching. Investigators have tried to identify strategies for early detection.

In American college swimmers a 10% incidence of burnout was reduced to zero by daily mood monitoring with a profile of mood state (POMS) questionnaire, and by reducing training when mood deteriorated and increasing it when mood improved.

A persistent rise in early morning heart rate despite rest is non-specific but does provide objective evidence that something is wrong. Underperformance is usually noticed too late and serial measurements of blood concentrations of haemoglobin and creatine kinase and of packed cell volume do not help. Good diet, full hydration, and rest between training sessions will help athletes tolerate hard training. Those with a full time job and other commitments will not recover as quickly as those who can relax after training. There are no objective tests to predict which athletes are going to break down during a period of hard training so adequate time has to be allowed for all of them to recover. Periodisation of training should permit this, with particular care at times of intensive interval training and hard monotonous training.

Management

Management of the overtraining syndrome

- Relaxation strategies and rest, with regular very light exercise
- Communication with the coach
- Strong reassurance that the prognosis is good

Overtrained athletes *v* patients with chronic fatigue

- Their primary presenting complaint is of underperformance, which is an objective measure of their condition
- They present earlier, are less severely affected, and recover more quickly
- The main stresses in their lives are exercise and competition, which can be controlled
- The main problem in rehabilitation is in holding them back, rather than having to encourage appropriate exercise

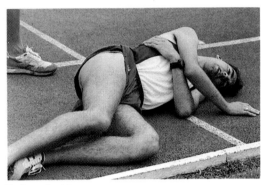

Fatigued athlete.

The treatment of any chronic fatigue syndrome requires a holistic approach, and athletes are no exception. Rest and regeneration strategies are central to recovery. Five weeks of rest appreciably improve both performance and mood state, and there is growing evidence that a very low level of exercise will speed recovery. Thus athletes must exercise aerobically (but not so hard that they cannot talk) for a few minutes each day and slowly build this up over many weeks. The level will depend on the clinical picture and rate of improvement, and recovery generally takes 6-12 weeks. Many make the mistake of trying to do a normal training session, suffering from severe fatigue for several days before partially recovering, and then doing it again. Cross training (playing another sport) may be the only way of avoiding the tendency to increase the intensity too fast.

Regeneration strategies are widely used in the old Eastern bloc countries, although there are no controlled trials of treatment. They consist of rest and relaxation with counselling and psychotherapy. Massage and hydrotherapy are used, and nutrition is looked at in detail. Large quantities of vitamins and supplements are given, although there is no evidence of their effectiveness. Any stresses outside sport are reduced as far as possible.

There is one report of the use of anabolic steroids (which are banned in athletes) in an attempt to speed recovery, but drugs are not generally of value unless depression is a major factor.

Athletes are often surprised at the performance they can produce after 12 weeks of extremely light exercise, and it is then that care must be taken not to increase training too fast. They need to train hard to go faster, but they must rest and recover completely at least once a week to benefit from all their hard work.

SUDDEN DEATH

W S Hillis, P D McIntyre, J Maclean, J F Goodwin, W J McKenna

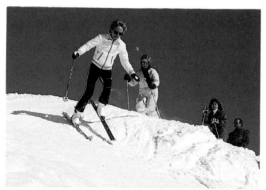

Skiing is a high intensity sport that makes moderate or high dynamic and static demands.

Most sudden deaths in sport are caused by cardiovascular conditions. The cardiovascular benefits of exercise are well established, and epidemiology studies suggest that long term exercise programmes may reduce the risk of sudden death. Increasing leisure time and facilities promote sports participation at all ages. A few people are at risk of serious arrhythmia or sudden death with exercise. The cause of death varies with the age of participants; congenital structural abnormalities occur in younger age groups and coronary artery disease in older age groups. Identifying such abnormalities makes prevention possible.

Sudden death in sport is uncommon, with an incidence of 2 cases per 100 000 subject years. Five in 100 000 athletes have a condition that might predispose them to serious cardiac problems, and of those at risk 10% (1 in 200 000) may die suddenly or unexpectedly. Considerable controversy exists about the cost effectiveness of screening all young people by examination before participation. Alternative views suggest targeting people with a family history of sudden death or premature coronary artery disease and educating all participants to see their doctors about even minor warning symptoms.

Some of the cardiac causes of sudden death will be suggested by symptoms and signs on clinical examination. The importance of others may be established only by detailed cardiological investigations including electrocardiography, chest radiography, echocardiography, doppler cardiography, and, rarely, cardiac catheterisation. Exercise testing is of major value and 24-48 hour tape electrocardiographic recordings may be required. Potentially serious symptoms such as syncope, pre-syncope, palpitation, chest pain, and undue dyspnoea should stimulate taking a detailed clinical history, making a detailed examination, and referring for cardiological investigation if appropriate. A family history of cardiac abnormality would suggest a hereditary basis.

Cardiac causes of sudden death

Coronary artery disease
Hypertrophic cardiomyopathy
Idiopathic concentric left ventricular hypertrophy
Congenital anomalies of coronary arteries
Aortic rupture
Right ventricular dysplasia
Myocarditis
Valvular disease
Arrhythmias and conduction defects
Congenital heart disease, operated or unoperated

General considerations

Classification of sports according to intensity and demands

A *High intensity*

1 *Moderate or high dynamic and static demands*

American football	Fencing	Running (sprinting)
Boxing	Ice hockey	Speed skating
Cross country skiing	Rowing	Water polo
Downhill skiing	Rugby	Wrestling

2 *Moderate to high dynamic, low static demands*

Badminton	Orienteering	Squash
Baseball	Race walking	Swimming
Basketball	Racket ball	Table tennis
Field hockey	Running (distance)	Tennis
Lacrosse	Soccer	Volleyball

3 *Low dynamic, moderate to high static demands*

Archery	Field events	Motor cycling
Auto racing	(jumping and	Sailing
Diving	throwing)	Ski jumping
Equestrian events	Gymnastics	Water skiing
	Karate or judo	Weight lifting

B *Low intensity, low dynamic and static demands*

Bowling	Curling	Shooting
Cricket	Golf	

By far the most common condition leading to sudden death during exercise, usually in those aged over 40, is coronary artery disease, including congenital abnormalities of the coronary artery tree. Death in younger athletes is rare but may be due to hypertrophic cardiomyopathy, right ventricular dysplasia, valvular heart disease such as aortic stenosis, and Marfan's syndrome.

Consensus discussions have suggested classification into high and low intensity sports, with further differentiation into those with major dynamic and static components.

Classification of sports according to danger of body collision

Contact sports	Non-contact sports	
American football	Auto racing	Ski jumping
Boxing	Bicycling	Water polo
Ice hockey	Diving	Water skiing
Karate or judo	Downhill skiing	Weight lifting
Lacrosse	Equestrian events	(increased risk if
Rugby	Gymnastics	syncope occurs)
Soccer	Motor cycling	
Wrestling	Polo	

Contact and non-contact sports must be distinguished and activities identified that may place a person in jeopardy if syncope occurs. Patients with a prosthetic cardiac valve should not participate in contact sports because of potential valve dehiscence during forceful chest contact and the risks of trauma in the presence of anticoagulant drugs. Most cardiovascular risk occurs with extreme exertion, such as marathon running, cross country running, skiing, basketball, football, hockey, and track sports.

Coronary artery disease

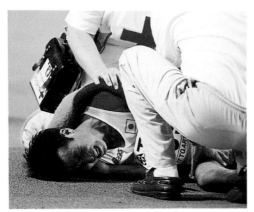

Marathon running is one of the most common causes of sudden death from coronary artery disease.

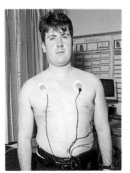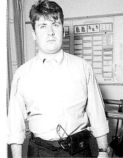

During 24-48 hour tape electrocardiography the contacts and leads are covered by clothing and the recorder fixed to the belt.

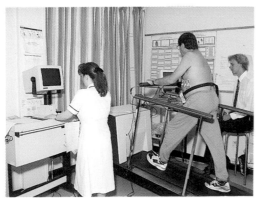

Exercise testing is useful to diagnose many cardiac disorders.

Coronary artery disease is the major cause of sudden death in older athletes (aged over 35). The risks are increasing as more middle aged and older people participate in organised competitive sport that requires vigorous physical exertion. During exercise metabolic and physical changes occur that lead to an increased risk. Even in conditioned older people, sudden death may be precipitated by occult coronary atheroma. Most deaths occur in running, competitive long distance racing, jogging, and other vigorous sports such as rugby, soccer, and squash.

History and risk factors

Previous symptoms suggestive of coronary atherosclerosis have often been recognised, and risk factors are frequently present, including smoking, a family history of myocardial infarction at under 55 years, hypertension, and hypercholesterolaemia. The victims are often perceived as being very fit and may have competitive personalities.

Pathology

In pathological studies, obstructive atheromatous coronary artery lesions are usually found, often associated with thrombus. The myocardium may show previous unrecognised healed infarcts.

Prevention

Extreme forms of conditioning, including marathon running, do not prevent severe atherosclerosis or sudden death. Education should be emphasised to increase awareness of warning symptoms such as chest pain, palpitation, or syncope. Severe exercise should be undertaken cautiously in patients aged over 40, particularly those with risk factors.

Diagnosis

The use of electrocardiograph stress testing to detect those at risk may have significant limitations. In addition, the incidence of false positives may be as high as 25% in sportsmen. People should be assessed in terms of their functional capacity and risk factors.

Degree of risk

Subjects with known coronary artery disease can be classified as being at low, moderate, or high risk by assessing left ventricular function, screening for evidence of reversible ischaemia, and comparing with the normal exercise capacity for age. Exercise testing may also detect ventricular arrhythmias or a reduced blood pressure response. High risk patients are those with decreased left ventricular systolic function at rest. Moderate risk patients are those with reduced exercise capacity for age, evidence of reversible ischaemia, ventricular tachycardia, or reduced systolic blood pressure. Low risk subjects with normal left ventricular function or without reversible ischaemia can participate in low intensity competitive sports, but those with moderate or high risk should be excluded. In patients who have had coronary artery bypass grafting or angioplasty serial assessment after the procedure should be undertaken.

Hypertrophic cardiomyopathy

Hypertrophic cardiomyopathy is the leading cause of sudden death in young athletes.

Anatomical abnormalities

A hypertrophied, non-dilated left ventricle exists but no history of predisposing diseases. The left ventricular chamber size is reduced and the muscular hypertrophy impairs diastolic filling. Left ventricular outflow tract obstruction may be secondary to hypertrophy of the subaortic septum or to systolic anterior motion of the mitral valve. There are predispositions to supraventricular and ventricular arrhythmias; ventricular tachycardia may lead to ventricular fibrillation.

Cause

Hypertrophic cardiomyopathy is inherited as an autosomal dominant condition that has a high degree of penetrance. When it is identified in an individual screening of all first degree relatives should be considered.

Symptoms

Patients may present with chest pain, palpitation, syncope, or breathlessness or may be asymptomatic. Abnormal cardiac findings may consist of a jerky or bisferiens pulse or an increased or double left ventricular apical impulse with a palpable fourth heart sound and a systolic murmur at the lower left sternal border that is decreased by squatting and increased by standing. The electrocardiogram is usually abnormal, although the findings may be non-specific. Cardiomegaly may be present on chest radiography but the diagnosis is made on echocardiography, which shows a small cavity and hypertrophy of the left ventricle, limited compliance, and limited diastolic filling.

Future exercise

The presence of cardiomyopathy should restrict people from engaging in strenuous dynamic or static sports, but those at low risk may follow a moderate exercise programme.

Differentiation from "athletic heart'"

Left ventricular hypertrophy in athletes is common as a normal response to training, but the ventricular wall is rarely more than 12 mm thick. A thickness of more than 16 mm is strongly suggestive of hypertrophic cardiomyopathy.

Prognostic factors for sudden death caused by hypertrophic cardiomyopathy

- Family history of sudden death
- Documented ventricular tachycardia
- Young age at onset of symptoms

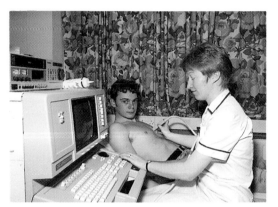

Echocardiography is the diagnostic test for hypertrophic cardiomyopathy.

Other causes

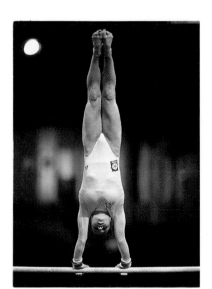

Gymnastics is a high intensity sport that makes low dynamic and moderate to high static demands.

Right ventricular dysplasia

Right ventricular cardiomyopathy or dysplasia has been reported as a cause of sudden death during sport, and may have a regional distribution. It is associated with fibrous, fatty replacement of the right ventricular myocardium, which is grossly dilated.

Congenital coronary artery abnormalities

Patients may present with symptoms of anginal pain, syncope with exertion, or even sudden death. Investigations should include a 12-lead electrocardiogram, a two dimensional echocardiogram to assess the position of origin of the left main coronary artery, and an exercise stress test.

Marfan's syndrome

Cardiovascular involvement gives mitral valve prolapse in almost all patients. If the syndrome is suspected on clinical appearance and by the presence of a family history the patient should be referred for regular echocardiography. β Blockers should be considered to retard the rate of aortic root dilatation and may be prescribed for patients with dilated aortic roots, and for those who have had aortic surgery.

Aortic stenosis

Symptoms from aortic stenosis of left ventricular failure, syncope, or anginal pain occur late. In those with a symptomatic, mild to moderate stenosis, participation may occur in low intensity sports (class B) or alternatively moderate static or dynamic demands (class A3).

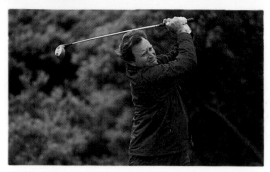

Golf is a low intensity sport with little danger of body collision.

Issues requiring further study include:

- Identifying causes of sudden death during physical exercise

- The appropriateness, cost, and practicality of cardiovascular screening of presumably healthy children and adolescents before they participate in sport and of other people before they continue or return to sport

- Counselling patients with known cardiac abnormalities about their levels of activity and about the risk and safety of specific sporting events

- Establishing guidelines for disqualification from competition

---

Mitral valve prolapse

The approach to mitral valve prolapse should be pragmatic. In the absence of symptoms and signs or associated lesions and with a negative family history, full sporting participation should be allowed. In the presence of palpitations, dizziness, or near syncope, both Holter monitoring and stress testing are invaluable for estimation of the mechanism of the symptoms. Associated problems that might exclude sporting activity include an associated prolonged QT syndrome or a family history of sudden death associated with a mitral valve prolapse.

Valve replacement

In patients who have had valvuloplasty or annuloplasty, contact sports should be avoided. Athletes with a prosthetic valve and normal cardiac function may engage in low intensity sports.

The pictures of the skier, marathon runner, gymnast, and golfer are reproduced with permission from Spectrum Colour Library, Allsport, Vandystadt, and Colorsport.

ASSESSMENT OF PHYSICAL PERFORMANCE

Clyde Williams

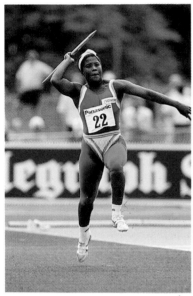

Fitness demands strength, speed, endurance, flexibility, and skill.

Measurable elements of fitness

- Strength   Isokinetic dynanometer
- Speed   Cycle ergometer
- Endurance   Treadmill (VO$_2$ MAX, %VO$_2$ MAX, blood lactate)
- Flexibility   Goniometers

VO$_2$MAX=maximum oxygen uptake, %VO$_2$MAX= relative exercise intensity.

Physical performance is mainly a function of an individuals's size, shape, sex, and age, but not entirely so. Success in sport at whatever level also depends on fitness. It is assumed, of course, that implicit in any definition of fitness is the absence of acute or chronic illness. Fitness is sport specific and in many sports it is also position specific. This "fitness for purpose" is a well accepted concept in sport, as reflected by the use of the word "fit" to describe, for example, successful runners, swimmers, gymnasts, and paraplegic athletes. Nevertheless, fitness for any sport has five common elements— strength, speed, endurance, flexibility, and skill. The relative contributions of each of these to the specific fitness demands of different sports are, of course, not equal. Training time devoted to each of these elements is therefore different between sports and depends on the level of participation. To a certain extent skill can compensate for poor fitness, but improved fitness allows skilful athletes to extend their performance by delaying the onset of fatigue.

Elite athletes develop fully each of the components of fitness as part of their preparation for competition at the highest levels. But even people participating in sport for recreation need to develop their fitness to enjoy their activities and to recoup the health benefits of exercise. All five elements contributing to fitness for sport also contribute to fitness for health. The one that must not be neglected is endurance. Rather than gold medals, the goal of most people taking exercise for health is the capacity to complete their daily round of activities with enough energy left over for recreation and relaxation. They are mainly interested in developing and maintaining good functional fitness; even so, their fitness can be assessed by the same procedures as are used for assessing elite athletes.

Endurance capacity

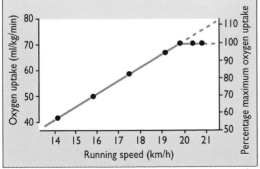

Relation between oxygen consumption and running speeds on a level treadmill to the point of exhaustion.

Prolonged submaximum exercise, irrespective of the form it takes, is tolerated because we can continue to supply working skeletal muscles with enough energy to cover their energy expenditure by the aerobic metabolism of fatty acids and carbohydrate. The energy produced by this metabolism is in the form of adenosine triphosphate (ATP), which has also been described as the "energy currency of life" because it is used to cover the cost of all cellular activities demanding energy.

Exercise comes to an end when either the muscles' limited carbohydrate stores (glycogen) are depleted or we become severely dehydrated. The exercise intensity we can tolerate for prolonged periods is dictated by several factors. The most important is the capacity of the cardiovascular system for oxygen transport. This is reflected by the amount of oxygen we use during heavy exercise lasting several minutes. As exercise intensity increases—for example, during walking or running on a treadmill or exercising on a cycle ergometer— the amount of oxygen we consume increases proportionally. A level of exercise is eventually reached at which we can no longer increase our rate of oxygen consumption; shortly thereafter we become exhausted.

Assessment of physical performance

Exercise protocol for assessing maximum oxygen uptake using a treadmill*

Treadmill slope (%)	Running time (min)	Expired air collection (min)
0	0-2	1¼-2
2	2-4	3¼-4
4	4-6	5¼-6
6	6-8	7¼-8
8	8-10	9¼-10
10	10-12	11¼-12
12†	12-14	13¼-14

*Running speeds were: men 13 km/h; elite men 14 km/h; women 11 km/h; elite women 12 km/h.
†Continues until the runner cannot complete 2 min.

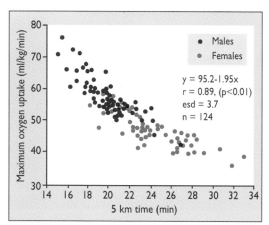

$y = 95.2 - 1.95x$
$r = 0.89, (p<0.01)$
$esd = 3.7$
$n = 124$

- Males
- Females

Relation between performance times during a 5 km track race and the maximum oxygen uptake of male and female runners. The anomalies between maximum oxygen uptake and performance times between runners can be explained by differences in their training status.

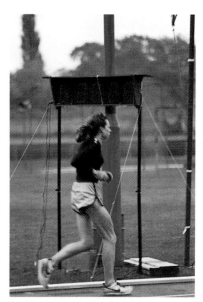

Endurance capacity is improved by an increase in capillary density in muscles.

Maximum oxygen uptake and relative exercise intensity

The highest rate of oxygen consumption is called peak or maximum oxygen uptake (VO_2MAX). We can describe any level of activity in terms of its oxygen cost as a proportion of an individual's maximum oxygen uptake. This description of exercise intensity is called the relative exercise intensity ($\%VO_2MAX$). Cardiovascular, thermoregulatory, and metabolic responses to exercise occur in proportion to the relative exercise intensity rather than the absolute rate of energy expenditure. This concept is particularly important when comparing different people's responses to exercise, whether they are athletes or people undergoing clinical examination.

Exercise protocol for assessing maximum oxygen uptake using a cycle ergometer

Rate of working (watts)		Cycling time (min)	Expired air collection (min)
Men	Women		
50	25	0-2	1¼-2
100	50	2-4	3¼-4
150	75	4-6	5¼-6
180	100	6-8	7¼-8
205	125	8-10	9¼-10
235	150	10-12	11¼-12
265*	175	12-14	13¼-14

*Continues until the cyclist cannot complete 2 min.

Variation in maximum oxygen uptake

Our maximum oxygen uptake is determined by age, height, weight, sex, and amount of daily physical activity. The larger its value the greater our exercise capacity. Therefore its assessment is essential in measuring performance. The values in active young women are 35-50 ml/kg/min, whereas the corresponding values in elite female endurance athletes are 55-70 ml/kg/min. Active young men have values of 50-65 ml/kg/min, whereas elite male athletes have values of 65-90 ml/kg/min.

In general people with high maximum oxygen uptakes have greater work capacities than those with lower values. Although training increases the maximum oxygen uptake, the improvement is not in proportion to the quality and duration of training. Nevertheless, exercise capacity is improved in proportion to the amount of training undertaken. Well trained athletes therefore perform better than those less well trained having similar maximum oxygen uptake values. Training status must be taken into account, along with maximum oxygen uptake, when describing the endurance capacity of an athlete.

Effect of training on metabolism

Endurance capacity, called aerobic fitness, is improved by a training induced increase in the densities of capillaries and mitochondria per muscle fibre. An increased number of mitochondria provides muscle with a greater capacity for aerobic metabolism of fatty acids and glycogen. Fat metabolism yields more ATP than the metabolism of an equivalent amount of glycogen, but this can be obtained only by aerobic metabolism. Therefore, these adaptations to endurance training allow skeletal muscle to use more fat to generate ATP and, in so doing, use their limited glycogen stores more sparingly. A training induced decrease in carbohydrate metabolism is reflected by lower blood and muscle lactate concentrations during exercise. One way of assessing endurance fitness therefore is to measure the changes in blood lactate concentrations during submaximum exercise of increasing intensity and thus identify the "lactate threshold" or "anaerobic threshold"—the exercise intensity at which the aerobic energy production (VO) is no longer sufficient to cover the demands of working muscles and so is complemented to anaerobic energy production.

Blood lactate concentrations and exercise intensity

Rather than attempt to detect the lactate threshold for athletes during routine testing, which would require an excessive amount of blood sampling, lactate reference values can be used. For example, blood lactate concentrations of 2 mmol/l and 4 mmol/l are used routinely for assessing changes in endurance or aerobic fitness. The rise in blood lactate concentration during exercise of increasing intensity is delayed after training, whereas after a prolonged period of inactivity or illness lactate concentrations increase significantly earlier in exercise. Routine assessments can be carried out without the need to perform exhausting exercise or to measure the maximum oxygen uptake because the results can be expressed as an exercise intensity at, for example, a lactate concentration of 2 mmol/l. This approach to assessing aerobic fitness is particularly attractive in a clinical setting when dealing with people whose health status does not permit exercise to exhaustion.

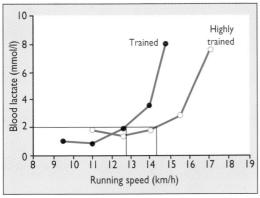

Blood lactate concentrations of two female runners of different training status but similar maximum oxygen uptakes during treadmill running over a range of submaximum speeds. The well trained runner was able to run faster before producing as much lactate as the less well trained runner.

Protocol for assessing blood lactate responses to submaximum exercise. The running speeds (mph) cover a wide range of submaximum exercise intensities (55%-90% Vo₂max) for most people

Running speed (mph)	Time (min)	Expired air collection (min)	Blood sampling (min)
6	4	3-4	3½-4
7	4	7-8	7½-8
8	4	11-12	11½-12
9	4	15-16	15½-16
10	4	19-20	19½-20

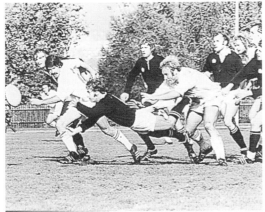

Rugby entails quick bursts of speed.

Ventilation rate and exercise intensity

The anaerobic threshold can also be assessed non-invasively by recording changes in ventilation rate during exercise of increasing intensity. The "ventilatory threshold" is the point at which there is a non-linear increase in ventilatory rate in relation to oxygen consumption. Although this approach to assessing aerobic fitness is attractive, the inflection point in the ventilatory responses to exercise is not always as detectable or sufficiently reproducible to recommend its measurement as routine procedure. In summary, a definition of endurance or aerobic fitness is that it is an individual's highest relative exercise intensity before producing a blood lactate concentration of 2 mmol/l. This definition allows the endurance fitness of everyone to be compared in a way that gives credit for the amount of training undertaken irrespective of age, sex, size, shape, or talent.

Speed

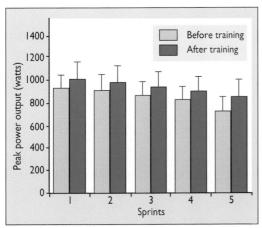

Mean (SD) peak power output values (watts) during repeated 6 s sprints with 30 s recovery before and after sprint training.

Absolute speed is a necessary prerequisite for runners striving for success in track races. But in many other sports the most important quality is the ability to perform brief sprints repeatedly with only short recovery periods. For example, soccer, rugby, cricket, and hockey are multiple-sprint sports. They require participants to perform brief sprints and to recover while continuing to run, jog, or walk. Fitness for the multiple-sprint sports is, therefore, best defined in terms of a player's ability to reproduce a series of sprints after only short recovery periods, rather than in terms of absolute running speed.

In many team games the pattern of activity is such that no one sprints for more than about five or six seconds and recovery periods are usually 30 seconds or more. When this activity pattern is reproduced on a non-motorised treadmill or cycle ergometer performance decreases after about five sprints. Improvements in performance after sprint training, however, are clearly seen and relatively easy to record. The external resistance on the cycle ergometer is the same as is used in the Wingate test (see below). This method provides a useful way of examining the strengths and weaknesses of individuals who participate in multiple-sprint sports.

Strength

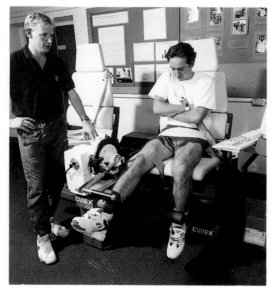

Testing muscle function using an isokinetic dynamometer.

Measuring muscle group strengths

Acquiring greater strength is a necessary part of developing fitness for most sports. Although the ability to lift heavier weights is unquestionably a measure of improved strength, the method does not allow the strength gains of individual groups of muscle to be assessed precisely. Recent developments in equipment for measuring isokinetic strength, however, provide the opportunity to make dynamic and precise measurements on a wide range of muscle groups during exercise of different intensities.

Testing the functional strength of the quadriceps, for example, requires angular velocities that are close to those experienced during free exercise. The functional angular velocities of the knee during walking have been reported to be about 233°/s, whereas during running the values increase to 1200°/s. The angular velocities used to test muscle performance of athletes should therefore be in the fast range, namely 300-450°/s. New versions of isokinetic muscle testing equipment can test in that range of movements. Repeated contractions provide an insight into the fatiguability of muscle groups and how training alters this particular aspect of muscle function. There are unfortunately no universally agreed isokinetic testing procedures for muscle function, mainly because in many laboratories the tests used are dictated by the design of isokinetic dynamometer.

To have records of muscle function of athletes when they are well trained and healthy is helpful not only as a means of following their adaptations to strength training, but also as invaluable reference during rehabilitation after injury or illness.

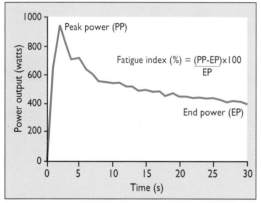

Power output values (watts) generated by an athlete while performing the Wingate anaerobic test on a cycle ergometer.

Measuring power output

In many sports the ability to generate power rapidly is more important than strength alone. Power in the context of sport may be regarded as the product of strength and speed. Peak power output can be measured safely, and accurately using a cycle ergometer and the Wingate test. The person performing the test must pedal as fast as possible against a resistive load, which is related to body weight (75 g/kg body weight), for 30 seconds. The onset and development of fatigue during that time can be recorded precisely when the ergometer is interfaced with a microcomputer.

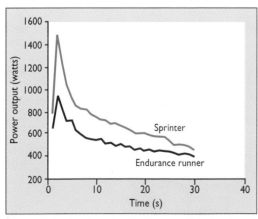

Power output values (watts) for a well trained sprinter and a well trained endurance runner while performing the Wingate anaerobic test on a cycle ergometer.

Histochemical analysis of muscle fibres

Muscle mass and its fibre composition dictates our ability to develop power, but muscle fibre composition is genetically predetermined. Fibre composition can be investigated from a histochemical analysis of muscle biopsy samples, but the relation between exercise performance and muscle fibre composition are not strong. Though histochemistry provides valuable information about energy demands of exercise and the adaptations to training, it is not a cost effective procedure for monitoring the progress of athletes in training.

Flexibility

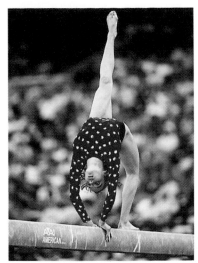

Flexibility allows the safe use of a wide range of movements

Flexibility is an essential part of training because it allows us to use a wide range of movements safely. In some sports such as gymnastics, flexibility is high on the list of training priorities. Coaches of such sports have their own methods of assessing improvements in flexibility. Comprehensive and reproducible assessment is difficult to achieve, however, because of the complex nature of movement. Nevertheless, carefully controlled measurements, albeit in limited ranges of movements, can be used to assess flexibility with a simple set of goniometers. It is particularly important that the measurements are standardised and that in longitudinal studies the same person performs all the measurements. The results can contribute useful information in assessing overall fitness when this strict code of practice is followed.

Conclusion

Fitness is a complex physiological characteristic that is difficult to describe comprehensively. Nevertheless, we can assess the central elements of fitness in reliable and reproducible ways. Through assessing athletes fitness we can extend health care by advising them on their ability to cope with the exercise demands of their chosen sport.

The photographs of the javelin thrower (Tessa Sanderson) and of the woman gymnast (Jackie Brady) were taken by Supersport Photographs.

NUTRITION, ENERGY METABOLISM, AND ERGOGENIC AIDS

Clyde Williams

Nutrition

Interest in the links between food and sports performance is not new. The physicians of antiquity advised the first Olympians about their training and pre-competition diets. The pre-competition meal is still the principal concern of those interested in the links between food and performance. There are, however, no "wonder foods," but there are nutritional strategies that can improve sports performance directly or indirectly through an improved capacity to train hard and recover quickly. These are effective only if athletes normally have well balanced diets, made up from a wide range of foods, and in sufficient quantity to cover their energy expenditures.

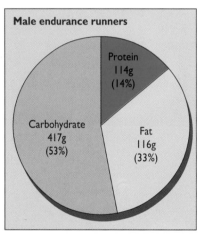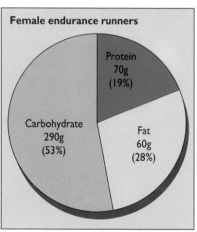

Composition of the daily food intake of 50 male distance runners to give 3200 kcal energy (left) and of 44 female distance runners to give 2000 kcal energy (right).

Proportions of dietary components

A healthy diet is one that derives at least 50% of its energy from foods containing carbohydrate, less than 35% from fats, and 12–15% from protein. However, of the whole population only endurance athletes (and vegetarians) have diets that match these recommendations. Because strength is an essential component of fitness many people believe that high protein diets contribute appreciably to strength gains. This is not the case. The daily protein requirement for most people is covered by an intake of about 1g/kg body weight. Those who train hard every day need slightly more, but only about 1·5–1·7 g/kg—far less than the large quantities of protein consumed by many strength athletes.

Amounts

"How much should I eat?" is as common a question from athletes as from less active people. The answer depends on their basal metabolic rates and their daily levels of physical activity. Basal metabolic rate (BMR) is the minimum amount of energy required to support life, and it accounts for 60% of our daily energy expenditure. It varies with age and sex and can be calculated from body weight. Physical activity level (PAL) is the type of activity performed in a day. The energy cost of each activity level is calculated by multiplying physical activity level by basal metabolic rate.

$$\text{Physical activity level (PAL)} = \frac{\text{Total energy expended during 24 hours}}{\text{Basic metabolic rate (BMR) over 24 hours}}$$

For example, people who are engaged in sedentary occupations have energy expenditures which can be met by an energy intake equivalent to about 1·55 times their basal metabolic rate whereas sports entailing prolonged heavy exercise require larger energy intakes. At the top end of the daily energy expenditure range are professional cyclists competing in long distance races. For example, in the Tour de France the professional cyclists have energy intakes of about 6500 kcal a day rising to about 9000 kcal/day during the alpine section of the race. They maintain energy balance during the whole of the three week race, sustaining an average physical activity level of about 3·3 times their basal metablic rate.

Formula for calculating basal metabolic rate (BMR) in kcal/day for either sex at different ages

Age (years)	BMR of males obtained from:	BMR of females obtained from:
10 to 17	17·5 × W+ 651	12·2 × W + 746
18 to 29	15·3 × W + 679	14·7 × W + 496
30 to 59	11·6 × W + 879	8·7 × W + 829

W=body weight in kg. BMR values obtained are in kcal/day.
(From the 1985 FAO/WHO/UNO report.)

Energy requirements for different levels of daily activity

	Type of daily physical activity level (PAL)		
	Light	Moderate	Heavy
Men	1·55 × BMR	1·78 × BMR	2·10 × BMR
Women	1·56 × BMR	1·64 × BMR	1·82 × BMR

(From the 1985 FAO/WHO/UNO report.)

Nutritional strategies

Two menus for high carbohydrate diets

Breakfast

Weetabix (4)	Baked beans on
Semi-skimmed milk	Thick sliced toast (3)
Crumpets (2) with honey	Low-fat spread (thinly spread)
Orange juice	Orange juice
Tea/coffee (preferably decaffeinated)	Tea/coffee (preferably decaffeinated)

Mid-morning snack

Malt loaf	Digestive biscuits (2)
Low -fat spread (thinly spread)	Banana
Diet squash (1 pint)	Low-fat milkshake

Lunch

French bread	Wholemeal hoagie
Lean ham	Lean beef
Reduced-fat Cheddar	Low-fat spread (thinly spread)
Low-fat spread (thinly spread)	Tomato, lettuce, cucumber
Pickles	Packet of "French fries" crisps
Low-fat rice pudding (eg) Mullerice	Low-fat fruit yoghurt
Pear	Diet squash/water
Diet squash/water	

Mid-afternoon snack

Apple and banana	Currant bun
Diet squash/water	Tea/coffee (preferably decaffeinated)

Dinner

Roast chicken	Pasta with lean ham, mushrooms, onion,
Mushrooms, onions, peas, and mixed	and cheese sauce
vegetables (stir-fried in a sweet and	(made with semi-skimmed milk and
sour sauce)	a cheese sauce packet mix)
Boiled basmati rice	Bread roll
Swiss roll and vanilla dairy ice-cream	Bread and butter pudding
Tea/coffee (preferably decaffeinated)	Tea/coffee (preferably decaffeinated)

Supper

Fruit 'n Fibre	Gingernut biscuits (5)
Semi-skimmed milk	Low-fat hot chocolate
Diet squash/water	

Energy 2944 kcal, of which:	Energy 2804 kcal, of which:
Protein (138 g) 19%	Protein (112 g) 16%
Fat 15%	Fat 22%
Carbohydrate 65%	Carbohydrate 62%

Carbohydrate before exercise

The strong link between glycogen depletion and fatigue during prolonged heavy exercise is well known. It is therefore not surprising that nutritional strategies have been developed to increase muscle glycogen stores before exercise. The most effective and acceptable method of carbohydrate loading is to decrease training during the three to four days before competition and increase the amount of carbohydrate-containing foods in each meal during this period. A daily intake of about 8-10 g carbohydrate per kg body weight is sufficient to increase muscle and liver glycogen stores before competition. Furthermore, a high carbohydrate meal eaten three to four hours before competition also helps to top up glycogen stores.

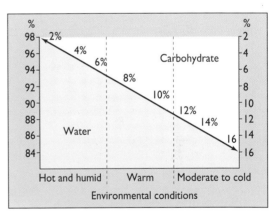

Guide to the recommended carbohydrate composition of fluids taken during exercise in different environmental conditions.

Fluid during exercise

Dehydration impairs performance during prolonged periods of activity and so fluid intake must also be part of nutritional strategies for competition and training. Dilute carbohydrate and electrolyte solutions are more effective as rehydrating agents than water alone because their electrolyte and glucose content increases the rate of water absorption across the small intestine. Exercise in hot humid conditions can be tolerated only as long as dehydration can be delayed. Sweat loss amounting to only 2–3% of body weight impairs performance, so high fluid intake is necessary to help delay the onset of dehydration.

Under these circumstances dilute glucose electrolyte drinks should be taken frequently. Under less extreme conditions there are also advantages to drinking solutions that supply more carbohydrate. Carbohydrate and electrolyte solutions that provide 30–50 g carbohydrate an hour increase endurance.

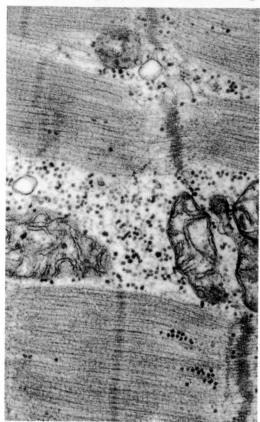

Electron photomicrograph of human muscle. The sample, obtained by percutaneous needle biopsy was taken before exercise to fatigue. The black dots are the glycogen granules dispersed between the myofibrils and mitochondria. Clear droplets of triglycerides, though not as abundant as the glycogen granules, are also visible.

Recovery after exercise

Speed of recovery from exercise depends on how quickly muscle glycogen can be replaced and fluid balance restored. Muscle glycogen resynthesis is most rapid immediately after exercise, so drinking a carbohydrate–electrolyte solution (or eating foods high in carbohydrate) immediately after exercise will produce the maximum rate of glycogen resynthesis. The optimum amount of carbohydrate is 1 g/kg body weight, which is achieved by drinking about a litre of a sports drink containing 6–7% carbohydrate. The overall carbohydrate intake during recovery over 24 hours should be equivalent to about 10 g/kg body weight. Delaying the consumption of carbohydrate for two to three hours after exercise reduces the rate of glycogen resynthesis and hence delays the return of endurance fitness. Furthermore, food intake during recovery must be prescribed because an ad libitum intake will not provide sufficient carbohydrate to replace muscle glycogen.

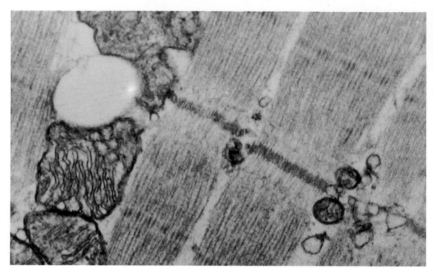

Electron photomicrograph of human skeletal muscle. The sample, obtained by percutaneous needle biopsy, was taken when the subject was fatigued after two hours of cycling. The absence of glycogen granules provides supportive evidence for the strong association between glycogen depletion and fatigue.

Nutritional supplements

Too many sports people are vulnerable to the advertising claims that nutritional supplements enhance performance. The most popular nutritional supplements are shown in the box, but there are many others which make claims without any supporting evidence.

Vitamins and minerals

Vitamin and mineral supplementation is a common practice among many sports people. However, there is no evidence to show that performance is enhanced after a period of supplementation of a well balanced diet with additional vitamins and minerals. But the assumption that athletes consume a diet containing a wide range of foods which provides sufficient energy to cover their energy expenditure is not always true. People who participate in sports with strict weight categories generally attempt to compete in a weight class that is lower than their normal training weight. Dieting to lose body weight to compete is as much a part of their sport as training. Low energy intakes and high energy expenditures pose the potential threat of nutrient deficiency. This is particularly true for women, who must pay particular attention to their iron and calcium intakes.

Popular nutritional supplements

- Vitamins

- Minerals

- Amino acids

- Carnitine

- Creatine

Amino acids

In addition to extra protein-containing foods, many strength athletes also supplement their diets with amino acids, especially those that they believe will stimulate an increased release of growth hormone, such as arginine. The growth hormone-releasing effect of these amino acids is far less than can be produced by exercise alone, but strength athletes and their coaches continue mistakenly to extol the performance benefits of amino acid supplementation.

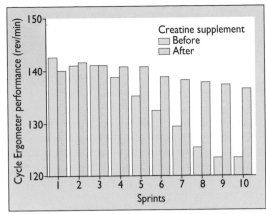

Influence of creatine supplementation on performance during 10 sprints, each of six seconds, on a cycle ergometer. (From Balsom PD, Ekblom B, Soderlund K, Sjodin B, Hultman E. Creatine supplementation and dynamic high-intensity intermittent exercise. *Scand J Med Sci Sports* 1993;**3**:143 9.)

Metabolic ergogenic aids

Metabolic ergogenic aids

- Caffeine
  (but effective amounts are banned by the International Olympic Committee)

- Bicarbonate
  (but effective amounts cause unpleasant reactions)

Conclusion

Carnitine

Carnitine has an essential role in fat metabolism. It is responsible for transporting fatty acids into mitochondria in skeletal muscles, where they undergo aerobic metabolism. The rationale for supplementing the diet with carnitine is that more fatty acid will be transported into mitochondria, which will result in increased fat metabolism. This in turn reduces the rate at which the limited glycogen stores are used for energy metabolism and so delays the onset of fatigue. Muscle has more than enough endogenous carnitine, however, so it is not surprising that carnitine supplementation has not been shown to improve human endurance capacity.

Creatine

In multiple-sprint sports the rate of ATP resynthesis is more important than the capacity for energy production. The rapid resynthesis of ATP occurs as a result of the contributions from the degradation of phosphrocreatine and from glycogenolysis. Performance during a series of maximum sprints, separated by recovery periods of no more than 30 seconds, decreases because there is not enough time for resynthesis of phosphrocreatine, even though there is sufficient glycogen to regenerate the ATP required. Creatine supplementation before exercise delays this decrease in performance by increasing the resynthesis of phosphrocreatine. The source of most of creatine is from foods containing meat or fish. However, creatine monohydrate is the supplement used and one gram is equivalent to the creatine content in 1 kg of fresh meat. In laboratory studies the effective dose of creatine is 20–30 g/day for five to six days. Creatine supplementation at this level increases the resting phosphrocreatine concentration but about half of the creatine intake is lost in the urine, hence the need for such high doses. Creatine is sold with the recommendation that two grams a day should be taken for a week before competition, it remains to be shown that this is an effective and, more importantly, a safe dose.

Caffeine

Caffeine is not a nutrient though it contributes to our diet through our consumption of coffee, tea, and soft drinks, Caffeine ingestion, in the form of four to five cups of coffee, increases the mobilisation of fatty acids and so offers working muscles an increased supply of this substrate. An increase in fat metabolism decreases the demands on the limited glycogen stores during prolonged exercise and so delays the onset of fatigue. Caffeine is also a stimulant of the central nervous system and this may also contribute to increased endurance capacity. Its disadvantage is that it is a diuretic and may contribute to dehydration. Furthermore, caffeine in the amounts that are effective in improving performance (several cups of coffee) is banned by the International Olympic Committee.

Bicarbonate

High intensity exercise lowers pH and this increase in acidity is associated with a reduction in anaerobic production of ATP and with a reduction in the rate of contractile activity. The ingestion of a bicarbonate solution (0·3 g/kg body weight) before heavy exercise increases plasma buffering capacity. Under these mildly alkalotic conditions lactic acid, or more correctly lactate and hydrogen ions, leave muscle cells more rapidly than under normal or acidic conditions. Running times in 400 and 800 metre track races are improved as a result of ingesting a bicarbonate solution two hours before competition. Nevertheless, the practice is not used widely probably because a common reaction to drinking a concentrated bicarbonate solution is abdominal distress and nausea.

Apart from appropriate training, a high carbohydrate diet and an adequate fluid intake are the essential elements in the formula for successful preparation for the participation in, and the recovery from, sport and exercise. A convincing case has yet to be made for supplementing a high carbohydrate, well balanced diet that is sufficient to cover daily energy expenditure.

DRUG MISUSE

David A Cowan

Sport, like most activities of civilised human endeavour, is regulated by rules. The uncivilised aspects are typically in direct contravention of those rules, and the intervention of the governing body is usually required to ensure that the rules are obeyed.

In top level sport the desire to win appears to be an essential ingredient for success. The use of ergogenic aids to enhance performance is an obvious choice. With the wide availability of many drugs that have the potential to enhance a competitor's sports performance, it is not surprising that such drugs are often taken by competitors with the sole aim of enhancing their performance. The sports world has decided that it wishes to control such drug taking.

Classes of drugs and drug administration

The act of taking substances that are banned by sports authorities is now usually known as doping. The rules of most governing bodies of human sport conform with those of the International Olympic Committee and consist of three main divisions:

(1) doping classes (which comprise the main groups of substances whose administration is banned by most international federations);

(2) doping methods (which include blood doping and pharmacological, chemical, and physical manipulation);

(3) classes of drugs subject to certain restrictions. This third division is a miscellaneous group of drugs either prohibited by certain sports—for example, alcohol in shooting—or is permitted only under specially controlled conditions—for example, corticosteroids, the use of which is permitted by certain routes of administration only.

The potentially harmful side effects caused by misuse of most of the doping substances argue in favour of controls to protect the health of competitors. Indeed the International Olympic Committee explains that its philosophy to control doping is intended to ban substances that might constitute a danger to the health of athletes when misused.

The International Olympic Committee bans classes of substances based on their chemical or pharmacological action. This reduces the possibility that non-listed "designer drugs" might be used to circumvent the rules, and hence the prospect of having competitions between the best pharmacologists rather than the best athletes.

How do athletes cope without a complete definitive list of banned substances? Great care is taken by organisations such as the British Olympic Committee, which, with the assistance of the Sports Council, issues many explanatory documents and gives lectures at training camps to the competitors under its care to ensure that they understand the doping rules and to warn them not to take any substance unless they are sure that it does not contravene the rules.

International Olympic Committee's Medical Commission's list of doping classes and methods
(September 1994)

I   *Doping classes*
(A) Stimulants
(B) Narcotics
(C) Anabolic agents
(D) Diuretics
(E) Peptide hormones and analogues

II   *Doping methods*
(A) Blood doping
(B) Pharmacological, chemical, and physical manipulation

III *Classes of drugs subject to certain restrictions*
(A) Alcohol
(B) Marijuana
(C) Local anaesthetics
(D) Corticosteroids
(E) β Blockers

The doping definition of the IOC Medical Commission is based on the banning of pharmacological classes of agents. The definition has the advantage that new drugs, some of which may be especially designed for doping purposes, are also banned.

Clinically necessary banned drugs

Sports competitors are subject to the same illnesses as other members of society and have the same right to normal medical treatment. What happens if a doctor's first choice of treatment conflicts with the rules of a sport? Fortunately this is a rare occurrence, not least because the International Olympic Committee has stated that it wishes to control drug misuse in sport while interfering with the normal therapeutic use of drugs as little as possible, and it takes this into account before banning a drug class. Nevertheless, consider, for example, the narcotic analgesics, which comprise one of the banned classes. A patient in great pain must be treated but pethidine, for example, might be expected to contravene the rules. Although technically this may seem to be the case, in practice it is not so, provided that the athlete does not immediately take part in

---

Some examples of narcotic analgesics are:

Dextromoramide	Dextropropoxyphene
Diamorphine (heroin)	Methadone
Morphine	Pentazocine
Pethidine	

. . . and related substances

Note: codeine, dextromethorphan, dihydrocodein, diphenoxylate, and pholcodine are permitted

TREATMENT GUIDELINES:

EXAMPLES OF PERMITTED AND **PROHIBITED** SUBSTANCES
(based upon International Olympic Committee Doping Classes 1993)

ASTHMA: ALLOWED—salbutamol inhaler, terbutaline inhaler

BANNED—products containing sympathomimetics (eg ephedrine, fenoterol, isoprenaline)

COUGH: ALLOWED—all antibiotics, steam and menthol inhalations, cough mixtures containing antihistamines

BANNED—products containing sympathomimetics (eg ephedrine, phenylpropanolamine)

DIARRHOEA: ALLOWED—diphenoxylate, loperamide, products containing electrolytes (eg Dioralyte, Rehidrat)

BANNED—products containing opioids (eg morphine)

HAYFEVER: ALLOWED—antihistamines, nasal sprays containing a corticosteroid or xylometrazoline, eye drops containing sodium cromoglycate

BANNED—products containing ephedrine, pseudoephedrine

PAIN: ALLOWED—aspirin, ibuprofen, paracetamol

BANNED—products containing opioids (eg dextropropoxyphene)

VOMITING: ALLOWED—domperidone, metoclopramide

CODEINE IS NOW PERMITTED FOR THERAPEUTIC USE

WARNING: THE ABOVE ARE ONLY EXAMPLES OF SUBSTANCES CURRENTLY PERMITTED OR PROHIBITED BY THE IOC. IF IN DOUBT CHECK WITH YOUR GOVERNING BODY OR WITH THE SPORTS COUNCIL. DOPING CONTROL UNIT 071 383 2244

REMEMBER—YOU ARE RESPONSIBLE

JUNE 1993

competition. Indeed, a doctor would probably not wish a patient to whom he or she has just administered pethidine to be competing. Patients requiring a milder analgesic may take codeine or any of the non-steroidal anti-inflammatory drugs, all of which are permitted.

Out of competition drug tests

Many governing bodies now conduct drug tests not only at competitions but also during the intervening periods. Action on finding a substance from one of the banned classes at an out of competition test is likely to be taken only if an anabolic or a masking agent is found. Thus any competitor requiring a drug from one of the banned classes, apart from the anabolic agents, may take the drug provided that they do not participate in competition. Indeed, refraining from the extremes of competition will probably greatly aid a patient's speedy recovery.

Some examples of stimulants are:

Amiphenazole	Amphetamines
Amineptine	Caffeine*
Cocaine	Ephedrines
Fencamfamine	Mesocarb
Pentylentetrazol	Pipradol
Salbutamol**	Terbutaline**

. . . and related substances

*For caffeine the definition of a positive result depends on the concentration of caffeine in the urine. The concentration in urine may not exceed 12 μg/ml
**Permitted by inhaler only and must be declared to the *relevant medical authority*.

Note: All imidazole preparations are acceptable for topical use (eg oxymetazoline). Vasoconstrictors (eg adrenaline) may be administered with local anaesthetic agents. Topical preparations (eg nasal or ophthalmological) of phenylephrine are permitted.

Stimulants

Asthma is probably the main condition for which treatment, at first sight, seems to contravene the doping rules. The β_2 adrenoceptor stimulants, the commonest treatment for asthma, are included under the stimulant doping class although two of them, salbutamol and terbutaline, are permitted provided that they are administered by inhalation. All other adrenoceptor stimulants are banned. However, the use of theophylline, aminophylline, or choline theophyllinate, as well as sodium cromoglycate or nedocromil sodium, is unrestricted. In addition, corticosteroids are permitted in certain circumstances.

Corticosteroids

The wide use of corticosteroids for their anti-inflammatory properties, and the restrictions placed on their use when administered by certain routes, makes this class of drugs worthy of special consideration. The International Olympic Committee bans the use of corticosteroids except for topical use (aural, ophthalmological, and dermatological); inhalation (for asthma or allergic rhinitis); and local or intra-articular injections. Any team doctor wishing to administer corticosteroids to a competitor intra-articularly or locally must give written notification to the International Olympic Committee medical commission. In the United Kingdom the Sports Council has devised a suitable form of notification where this is required by a governing body. Of course, severe asthma can be fatal and must be treated promptly. Intravenous hydrocortisone or oral prednisolone should be given without delay.

The application of corticotrophin is considered to be equivalent to the oral, intramuscular, or intravenous application of corticosteroids. However, corticotrophin is no longer available commercially and both it and its synthetic analogue, tetracosactrin, are probably of value only to test adrenocortical function.

International Olympic Committee's Medical Commission's rules on antiasthma drugs

Drug class	Banned	Permitted (by inhalation only)
Corticosteroids	All oral, intramuscular (depot), or intravenous preparations	Budesonide (Pulmicort) Beclomethasone (Becotide)
Selective β adrenoceptor stimulants	All oral, depot, or intravenous preparations and fenoterol (Berotec) inhalation	Salbutamol (Ventolin) Terbutaline (Bricanyl)
Non-selective adrenoceptor stimulants	Ephedrine Isoprenaline (Medihaler)	
Antimuscarinic bronchodilators	None	Ipratropium (Atrovent) Oxitropium (Oxivent)
Cromoglycate preparations	Cromoglycate with isoprenaline (Intal compound)	Cromoglycate (Intal) Nedocromil (Tilade)
Theophylline	None	

Some examples of anabolic androgenic steroids

Clostebol	Fluoxymesterone
Metandienone	Metenolone
Nandrolone	Oxandrolone
Stanozolol	Testosterone

. . . and related substances

Some examples of β₂ agonists

Clenbuterol
Salbutamol
Terbutaline
Salmeterol
Fenoterol

. . . and related substances

Some examples of diuretics

Acetazolamide	Bumetanide
Chlorthalidone	Ethacrynic acid
Furosemide	Hydrochlorothiazide
Mannitol	Mersalyl
Spironolactone	Triamterene

. . . and related substances

Some examples of β blockers

Acebutolol	Alprenolol
Atenolol	Labetalol
Metoprolol	Nadolol
Oxprenolol	Propranolol
Sotalol	

. . . and related substances

Conclusion

Further information on substances currently permitted or prohibited can be obtained by telephoning the Doping Control Unit on:

0171 383 5667 *or*
0171 383 5411
0171 383 2244

Doping Control Unit, Sports Council, Walkden House, 3-10 Melton Street, London NW1 2EB

Anabolic agents

This group includes the androgenic-anabolic steroids, the recognised therapeutic indications for which are very limited. In men the anabolic steroids testosterone (as one of its esters) and mesterolone may be used to treat androgen deficiency. In addition, testosterone is currently being evaluated for use as a male contraceptive. Its active metabolite, dihydrotestosterone, although not currently licensed in the United Kingdom, is also used to treat androgen deficiency. Its use, however, and that of any of the androgens is not permitted in sport. There is probably no real indication for the use of androgens in women who are well enough to compete, and women taking androgens, like men, may not take part in competitive sport.

Clenbuterol is marketed in Germany as a β₂ adrenoceptor stimulant but is also known to have appreciable protein accretion activity in animals. Its use is therefore not permitted under either the stimulant or the anabolic agent categories.

Human chorionic gonadotrophin in men leads to an increased rate of production of endogenous androgenic steroids and is considered to be equivalent to exogenous testosterone. Its use is therefore banned under the peptide hormone and analogues category.

Peptide hormones and analogues

As well as human chorionic gonadotrophin and corticotrophin, human growth hormone and erythropoietin are also banned. Doctors are unlikely to consider giving either of these substances to patients who are competing athletes. However, an awareness that athletes would consider administering these drugs to themselves may be helpful should a doctor encounter a request to prescribe them.

Diuretics

Diuretics are sometimes misused to reduce weight quickly in sports that have weight categories and also to reduce the concentration of drugs in urine to minimise detection of drug misuse. The International Olympic Committee considers that rapid reduction of weight in sport cannot be justified medically. Health risks are involved in such misuse because of possible serious side effects. It therefore bans the use of diuretics. For sports with weight classes, its medical commission reserves the right to obtain urine samples from the competitors at the time of weighing in. Female athletes with pre-menstrual tension whose doctors are considering prescribing a mild diuretic can probably take the tablets without failing an out of competition drug test, provided that they are not soon to take part in competition. Only the stronger diuretics, such as the loop diuretics, are likely to have an effect great enough for them to be considered as masking agents.

β blockers

The medical commission considers that there is a wide range of effective alternative preparations available to control hypertension, cardiac arrhythmias, angina pectoris, and migraine. The continued misuse of β blockers in some sports in which physical activity is of no or little importance, has led the commission to reserve the right to test competitors in sports that it deems appropriate. These are unlikely to include endurance events, which necessitate prolonged periods of high cardiac output and large stores of metabolic substrates, for which β blockers would severely decrease performance capacity. There is no restriction on the use of angiotensin converting enzyme inhibitors or calcium channel blockers to treat hypertension. Similarly, there is no restriction on the use of other drugs, such as ergotamine or sumatriptan, for migraine.

This short chapter tries to answer some of the commonly raised questions. However, how do practising doctors cope without a complete definitive list of banned substances? The *British National Formulary* now carries details of a help line for doctors who need guidance about whether drugs they are considering offering to patients who also compete in sport might be banned from that sport. The responsibility for the treatment may be a partnership between doctor and patient, but in the eyes of sports authorities, which consider participation a privilege, the responsibility for adhering to the doping rules usually rests solely with the athlete.

TEAM MEDICAL CARE

Donald A D Macleod

The medical team

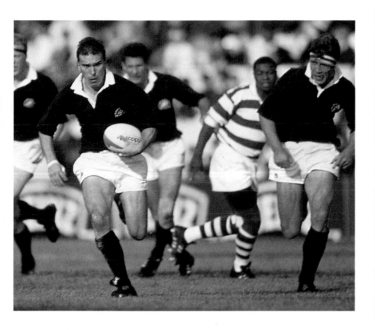

Objectives

Preparation for performance

- Helping to enhance fitness, skill, and co-ordination while minimising the risks of overtraining or injury
- Advice about diet, vaccinations, travel, jet lag, acclimatisation, insurance

Prevention of injury or illness

- safety of playing environment
- protection from inclement weather
- availability of first aid and rescue facilities appropriate to the activity

Management of injury or illness

- based on well recognised patterns associated with sport such as knee injuries, cuts, viral illnesses, etc, but always be prepared for a crisis. Every sport is associated with risk

Research, audit, and documentation

- to enhance player safety and performance

A doctor and chartered physiotherapist usually make up the staff involved in the medical care of a team but this can vary between sport and may include a masseur or sports scientist. The essential difference between team medical care and colleagues providing services at an event or to a governing body in sports is the very special, professional but highly committed and enduring relationship that arises as the result of being part of the inner circle of players, coaches, selectors, and the team manager.

The medical team aims to underpin the playing team and must therefore be an integral part of the inner circle if they hope to provide the highest standards of occupational health.

The medical team cannot expect to be omnicompetent in the increasingly sophisticated world of sports medicine and sports science. The team will require appropriate facilities as well as a network of specialist advisers.

The medical team shares the highs and lows of their team's successes and failures as well as working with individuals to help them achieve their peak performance. To this end, the medical team should set realistic objectives.

In most sport the medical team may well be giving their professional advice on a voluntary basis but this does not allow for any lowering of professional standards of practice—players are not experimental preparations or second class citizens.

The performing life of an athlete may be very short and the pressures to compete are intense but the medical team must be objective about the individual player/patient while remaining enthusiastically committed to the players and their realistic goals.

The medical team must demonstrate many personal and professional skills if they are to win a respected position in the inner circle.

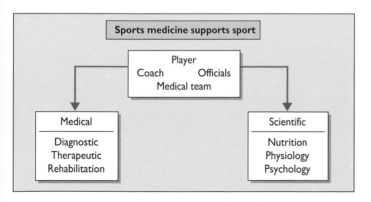

Personal attributes

Members of the medical team must work together to fulfil their respective roles, clarifying lines of communication. There is no place for prima donnas in the medical team. Mutual respect and support are essential.

Knowledge—Sports medicine is no longer a hobby. Doctors involved in sport must be prepared to stand up to peer review on the basis of their knowledge and experience—as shown by passing an exam such as the Joint Scottish Royal Colleges Diploma in Sports Medicine.

Enthusiasm for the sport and participants, irrespective of their level of involvement, and for the specialty of sports medicine, is essential.

Availability—If the players and coaches are out working on a foul night in the middle of winter, the medical team should be there with them. Medical staff should also be available in and out of season, as well as when training and playing; there is no closed season.

Support, tolerance and understanding are needed from family and colleagues.

Knowledge of the players as patients should be on a professional basis (with interview and examination): (1) before a sport such as scuba diving, boxing; (2) before an event, usually for insurance purposes; and (3) after an injury or illness, when the medical team must be completely honest about diagnosis, treatment, rehabilitation, and return to competition.

Winning the players' trust is needed to ensure they will respect medical staff judgment even in the most difficult circumstances—for example, in withdrawing from a competition or sport.

Knowledge of the game—The medical team must understand the rules of the game and not be party to attempts to win at all costs by condoning the "VD" (violence or drugs) of sport by manipulating standards of clinical practice to give the player a professionally unwise chance of competing when not fit. Medical staff should document injuries and illness occurring in the game and use this information to promote player safety as well as appropriate treatment protocols.

Knowledge of officials—If it is to fulfil its role in the inner circle, the medical team must work with a wide range of officials. These include coaches, selectors, and managers, referees, and administrators. They should also clarify the exact professional relationship between the players, their general practitioners, and officials. In contacts with the media and the public the medical team should maintain clinical confidentiality and ethical standards, with no discussion of patient details without permission.

Drugs and treatment methods

The most valuable drugs or treatments prescribed by any member of the medical team are time and honesty. Most players will talk themselves out of many minor injuries or illnesses that have been precipitated by stress, underperformance, training loads, and competitions. Individual and team morale can often be gauged in the medical team room.

Care of acute soft tissue injuries

Minimise tissue disruption
- Rest injured part
- Ice
- Compression
- Elevation
- Non-steroidal anti-inflammatory drugs

} for 36 hours

Accurate diagnosis
- Requires serial examination at the time of injury and over the following 72 hours
- Investigations are rarely relevant in most common injuries but modern scanning techniques can be helpful

Definitive treatment
- Give nature a chance (the capillary buds, macrophages, and fibroblasts require time to complete the process of healing)
- Minimise medical interference but ensure appropriate specialist support is available by establishing networks
- Give physiotherapy
- Rehabilitate to prevent recurrence
- Maintain overall fitness and skill

Players must always be encouraged to take responsibility for their own treatment and rehabilitation programmes. The medical team should never act as a crutch to support lame ducks; players deserve the benefits of self respect and independence.

The treatments used to ease minor injuries or illness, whether acute of chronic, must not be used in a random, poorly researched, illogical, or blunderbuss way.

Overuse and chronic soft tissue injuries are often a challenge to the medical team, requiring considerable experience and ingenuity to relieve the problem, working closely with the player and the coach.

Underperformance by an athlete is a topic requiring detailed medical knowledge.

The team doctor must always clarify with a player the ethical relationship between the player, the coach or selector, and the team manager. When appropriate, close liaison with the player's own general practitioner is essential.

Drugs

The drugs carried in a medical bag are the standard general practitioner or accident and emergency prescriptions that will cover the range of injuries, infections, and illnesses encountered in sport, ranging from sprains and strains, skin fungal infections, and dyspepsia. The role of short courses of non-steroidal anti-inflammatory drugs and local anaesthetic with steroid injections in sports requires objective assessment of their value. Team doctors must never prescribe any drug that is banned by the International Olympic Committee or the regulations applying to the sport with which they are involved.

The photograph was supplied by the Scottish Rugby Union.

BENEFITS OF EXERCISE IN HEALTH AND DISEASE

P H Fentem

P H Fentem

Recommendations of the Royal College of Physicians

- There is now good evidence of many physical and psychological benefits available to the population from regular exercise which should be recognised by all those involved in health care
- The habit of taking regular recreational exercise is best started in childhood and should be continued into middle age and where possible into old age because exercise helps to make the most of diminishing physical capacity
- Doctors should ask about exercise when they see patients, particularly when they come for routine health checks, and should be aware of and advise on suitable exercise programmes
- The value of exercise for patients with a wide range of disorders should be considered and advice given on the type and extent of activity to be undertaken
- Doctors should be aware of the relevant risks that exercise may pose for individual patients. When exercise is of suitable intensity for the individual, is taken regularly and with sensible precautions, the benefits greatly outweigh any risks

---

The claim that individual participation in adequate amounts of regular physical activity can improve health and prevent disease is fully justified. The scientific evidence is based on many studies—epidemiological, clinical, and physiological. A working party of the Royal College of Physicians, convened in 1989, examined this evidence, recognised its importance, and based a series of recommendations on it.

Coronary heart disease and stroke are identified as key priorities in the white paper, *Health of the Nation*. In these two conditions individual risk is dramatically reduced by a change in lifestyle and an increase in physical activity. Other important benefits must not be overlooked. The list is extensive but falls into four categories: enhancing function, maintaining reserve capacities, preventing disease, and ameliorating the effects of age and chronic disease.

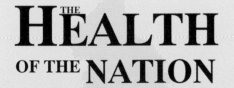

Beneficial effects on heart disease or stroke should result from:

- Stopping smoking
- Reducing consumption of saturated fatty acids and sodium
- Reducing alcohol consumption
- Increasing physical activity

The task of achieving appropriate changes in lifestyle and of successfully promoting physical activity is formidable. Primary health care teams have been given an important role in implementing health promotion strategies. *Better Living—Better Life*, prepared by the Joint Working Group on Health Promotion and sent to all general practices last year, is an important resource. It contains the background, ideas for action, and advice about how to motivate patients and should prove indispensible for those contracting to undertake this work.

Recognition of the importance of the benefits conferred by regular physical activity has been slow to develop among those concerned with health care in the United Kingdom. According to the Allied Dunbar national fitness survey, three quarters of the general public (adults over 16 years of age) understand that exercise confers important health benefits but not what that means.

Functional changes and improvements achievable through exercise

Skeletal muscle functions enhanced by exercise

- Metabolic capacity and nutrient blood supply
—Increases stamina
—Ameliorates effects of age and chronic disease, including coronary heart disease

- Strength and contractility
—Increases capacity for work and exercise
—Reduces risk of injury
—Ameliorates effects of muscle disease

The health benefits of exercise are explicable in terms of favourable physiological, psychological, and biochemical changes and improvements in function. Their scope is greater than has been supposed. Motivating sedentary people to pursue these benefits is not straightforward. They are reluctant to undertake even moderate exercise, and they become immediately aware of their limited tolerance for physical work and the discomfort that it provokes. It takes several weeks of regular exercise to see an improvement in their capacity for effort and for there to be a training effect.

Tendon and connective tissue functions enhanced by exercise

- Strength
- Supportive function
- Joint stability
—Reduces risk of injury especially with age and muscle disease

Joint functions enhanced by exercise

- Lubrication
—Avoids limitation of movement
- Range of movement
—Limits effects of degenerative arthritis
- Maintenance of flexibility

The objective should be to take enough regular exercise to improve or maintain stamina, to strengthen muscles, and to improve or maintain the range of joint movement. To improve stamina the effort needs to be somewhat greater than that to which the person is accustomed. This means that those who have previously been sedentary will show an improvement in some capacities even with a low intensity of exercise. The degree of improvement also depends on the duration and frequency of the activity. If an increased level of activity is sustained then the cumulative effects of training build up over many months. These decline again if the exercise is discontinued. Harmful effects are unlikely, provided that the intensity of exercise is increased gradually. A variety of activities is important because the changes induced in skeletal muscles by training, increased vascularity, and improved biochemistry are specific to the muscles used and how they are used. Guidelines for the safe prescription of exercise will be published later in the series.

After training people of any age can work harder, longer, and with less effort than previously: there is a reduced sense of effort for any given task. This is true for everyone and for all age groups including elderly people. A dose-response relation is apparent.

Prevention of coronary heart disease and stroke

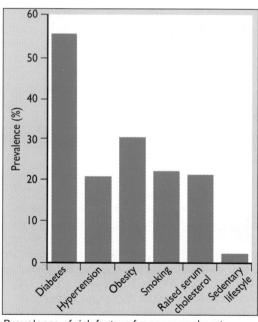

Prevalence of risk factors for coronary heart disease and stroke. Sedentary lifestyle means no or irregular physical activity (fewer than three times a week or less than 20 minutes per session (less than level 2 of Allied Dunbar national fitness survey)).

Reducing the risk of heart attack and stroke

A sedentary lifestyle is an independent risk factor for coronary heart disease and stroke. High amounts of habitual physical activity reduce the individual risk for both conditions. The evidence derives from prospective and retrospective epidemiological studies. Fewer studies have been undertaken of the risk reduction of stroke, but the results lead to similar conclusions. The need for measures to raise the amount of habitual physical activity by the general public is as pressing as the need for ways to combat raised blood cholesterol concentration, raised arterial blood pressure, and smoking. A high proportion of the public stands to benefit from increased exercise because so many people currently take none. Physical activity is likely to be protective through a combination of effects on other recognised risk factors, on metabolic and regulatory processes, on the profile of cholesterol and blood lipid concentrations and clotting factors, possibly on arterial blood pressure, and through its role in weight reduction.

What matters is that people of all ages, but especially those in middle age, currently engage in regular physical exercise of vigorous or moderate intensity and continue to do so. As to the amount of exercise, brisk walking every day will have an effect. Two to three kilometres of brisk walking on three days each week is sound advice on the available evidence. Whether more frequent but shorter walks will suffice provided that the total is 8-16 km each week is unclear, but it seems a reasonable assumption. A recent recommendation by the American College of Sports Medicine, the Centers for Disease Control and Prevention (CDC), and the President's Council on Physical Fitness and Sports takes this approach saying:

Every American adult should accumulate 30 minutes or more of moderate-intensity physical activity over the course of most days of the week. Because most Americans do not presently meet the standard described above, almost all should strive to increase their participation in moderate and/or vigorous physical activity.

This represents a definite shift in emphasis towards promoting physical activity of moderate rather than vigorous intensity and towards increased frequency of participation, at least five times a week rather than three times.

Prevention of mild or moderate systemic arterial hyptertension

High amounts of habitual exercise are a factor in determining the likelihood of arterial hypertension developing in previously healthy normotensive men and women.

Regular physical activity reduces both systolic and diastolic arterial blood pressure. Relatively small numbers of adults with mild or moderate or labile systemic arterial hypertension have been studied, but those who undertook regular physical activity experienced a reduction in arterial blood pressure of, on average, 10/8 mm Hg. This reduction is certainly therapeutically important but current opinion suggests that, for the time being, exercise should be considered an adjunct to other treatment.

American recommendations

- Women to walk 2 miles in <30 minutes at least 3 days a week
- Men to walk 2 miles in <27 minutes at least 3 days a week
- Or 2 miles in 30-40 minutes 6 days a week
- Or a total of 2 miles (3 km) each day in 3 periods of 10 minutes

Cardiac rehabilitation

One aim of rehabilitation must be to increase the patient's general capacity for physical work. A programme of regular exercise will achieve this improvement and by so doing will actually reduce the work which the heart must perform during physical effort. Thus regular exercise spares the heart by reducing the amount of work it has to perform. This comes about in two ways. Because the heart beats less frequently with improvement in aerobic fitness the energy requirement of the heart muscle is reduced. Because the systemic arterial blood pressure also falls this too reduces the workload on the heart muscle. As an extension of this, maximal myocardial performance is increased, allowing more exercise to be taken than before. Active cardiac rehabilitation is physiologically sound.

Current regular exercise has a significant place in secondary prevention of coronary heart disease and stroke. Despite some increase in the hazard for individual patients while they are exercising the benefits greatly outweigh these risks. Patients need not be advised against regular walking and exercise after stroke or heart attack, rather they should be encouraged and helped to increase the intensity of their exercise cautiously. Increments should be made every 8 or 10 weeks, provided that the patient complies with previous advice.

Prevention of sudden death in coronary heart disease

The risk factors for sudden death are similar to those for other manifestations of coronary heart disease. Thus it is not surprising that the general risk is moderated by regular exercise. The question of the risk of death or accident during a bout of exercise will, because of its importance, be considered in more detail later in the series.

Claims have not been substantiated that exercise leads to an increase in the diameter of coronary arteries, to formation of collateral vessels after a block or partial block of any of the three main coronary arteries, or to a decrease in the sensitivity of coronary arteries to spasm.

Cardiovascular functions enhanced by exercise

- Cardiac performance/myocardial work
—Ameliorates the effects of age and chronic disease, including coronary heart disease
- Arterial blood pressure regulation
—Reduces blood pressure in mild hypertension and attenuates age dependent rise
- Electrical stability of heart muscle
- Cardiovascular and sympathoadrenal response to acute exercise
—Reduces risk of cardiac arrhythmias and probably of sudden death

---

Prevention of other diseases

Functions of skeleton enhanced by exercise

- Maintenance of bone mass
- Adjustment of structure to load
—Prevents osteoporosis and fractures

Osteoporosis

Weight bearing exercise prevents osteoporosis. Regular physical exercise is one of several possible strategies for combating osteoporosis and the consequential fractures of the hip, wrist, and vertebrae. Habitual physical activity maintains and increases the mineral content of the skeleton. The effect is apparent at every age.

Skeletal bone mass increases during childhood and adolescence. The greater the peak bone mineral density at the end of growth the longer it will take to reach the fracture threshold in later life. Active children and young adults have denser bones than children who take little exercise.

After adolescence the bone density plateaus and then, after the fourth decade, decreases. At any age bone density is higher in men than in women. The rate of decline in bone mass is similar in both middle aged men and women except that in women the rate of loss accelerates for several years immediately after the menopause. These differences are sufficient to explain why elderly women reach the fracture threshold more often.

Habitual physical activity with weight bearing will halt or reverse the decline in density at any age. Women of all ages from 20 to 80 who exercise at least three times each week have a higher bone density than those who are sedentary.

Non-insulin dependent diabetes mellitus

Habitual physical activity prevents non-insulin dependent diabetes mellitus. Laboratory studies had shown that exercise can increase insulin sensitivity and improve glucose tolerance, which offers an explanation for the favourable effect of activity on the prevalence of this condition. These biochemical changes benefit obese people, especially those with non-insulin dependent diabetes.

Good metabolic control can still be achieved by young diabetic patients who participate in sport because exercise, even vigorous exercise, leads to a predictable reduction of the exogenous insulin requirement.

Metabolic functions enhanced by exercise

- Control of body weight
—Regulates energy balance
—Prevents obesity related disease and excessive weight gain
- Insulin sensitivity and carbohydrate tolerance
—Improves carbohydrate tolerance
—Ameliorates late onset diabetes
- Lipid and lipoprotein metabolism
—Prevent coronary heart disease and possibly stroke
- Inhibition of blood clotting processes
—Counters acute precipitants of cardiac arrest

Psychological functions enhanced by exercise

- Mood
  —Reduces mild anxiety and depression
- Self esteem
  —Influences mood favourably
- Psychomotor development
  —Contributes to the quality of care for those with learning difficulties
- Memory
  —Can improve memory in elderly people
- Calmness
  —Can ameliorate stress related conditions

Cancer

Several recent epidemiological studies have observed that physically active people are less likely than those who have a sedentary lifestyle to develop breast and colon cancer.

Minor mental illness

Improvements have been observed in patients with mild depression and anxiety, raising questions about its value as an adjunct to other measures in the management of minor mental illness. Because the physiological changes with regular exercise extend the range of activities that can be undertaken with confidence and ease, some of the psychological benefits are possibly linked to an improved general feeling of wellbeing. Other favourable effects have been noted.

Prevention of progressive incapacity

Assessing habitual physical activity: Allied Dunbar national fitness survey

Level*	No of occasions of type of activity
5	≥12, vigorous
4	≥12, mix of moderate and vigorous
3	≥12, moderate
2	5-11, at least moderate
1	1-4, at least moderate
0	None

*Based on 20 minute occasions of vigorous or moderate or mixed intensity.

Physical inactivity as cause of avoidable disability

The prevalence of physical disability attributable to age or chronic disease is high. Inactivity compounds the effects of these disabilities; this needs to be recognised because inactivity is often reversible but not inevitable and is common at all ages. The results of the Allied Dunbar national fitness survey showed that one third of men and two thirds of women would find it difficult to sustain walking at a moderate pace (about 3 mph up a 5% slope). The survey showed that people's rates of participation in active sports and exercise are low. About one out of every six people is sedentary and reported no activities whatsoever of a duration and intensity likely to benefit his or her health.

Benefits for disabled and elderly people

In general, people who are old and people with a disability are particularly prone to the deleterious effects of inactivity. Any illness or transient incapacity accelerates the deterioration. The vicious cycle of inactivity leading to deterioration and progressive loss of fitness and capacities occurs rapidly and reflects closely the time scale of the vascular and biochemical deterioration in unused muscles. For these reasons rehabilitation must always be active and enthusiastic and inactivity must not be accepted as normal.

Exercise offers important benefits to elderly people, enabling them to maintain a reasonable degree of fitness for the tasks of daily living, reducing handicap, and helping to avoid or delay the necessity for institutional care. Because exercise increases energy expenditure it tends to increase the overall dietary intake, including the intake of substances which occur in small amounts. Thus the minimal requirement of elderly people for vitamins is more likely to be met. Regular physical movement can play a part in avoiding constipation and associated flatulence.

Exercise to improve muscle strength when successful brings confidence in negotiating steps and other barriers. Some elderly people with rheumatoid arthritis and others with muscular dystrophy report an increased freedom: they can to go out of the house and travel independently on public transport. People with rheumatoid arthritis may return to work after previously giving up their jobs because of their health. Physically active wheelchair users have a lower rate of absence from work and fewer admissions to hospital than inactive colleagues. Both motor skills and the speed at which manual work is performed improve in people with intellectual impairment.

In some conditions symptoms are ameliorated during exercise programmes. Admittedly, exercise will never replace function lost through impairment, but the evidence suggests that people with rheumatoid arthritis experience a decrease in the number of painful or swollen joints and the degree of pain and swelling. Consequent conditions and further deterioration may be prevented, delayed, or reduced by regular exercise. Joint contractures are prevented in children who walk rather than use a wheelchair. Exercise in the upright position reduces calcium loss after a spinal cord injury. Wheelchair athletes have fewer pressure sores and kidney complications than sedentary wheelchair users. Children with cystic fibrosis who are active have fewer respiratory infections than those who are not.

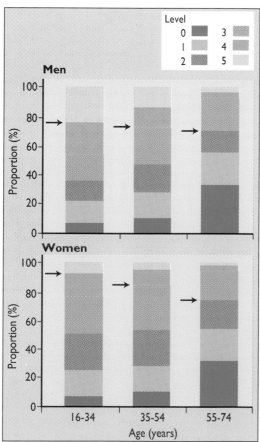

Proportion of respondents in each of six levels of Allied Dunbar national fitness survey. Arrows show targets for people of different ages.

Who needs advice about exercise?

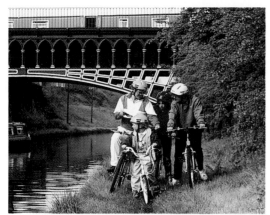
Cycling with the family is one enjoyable way to exercise.

Almost all those over 50, however sedentary or whatever their health problem, can benefit from physical activity provided that progress is slow and cautious

Most people do not regularly take exercise during leisure time or at work sufficient to benefit their health; the degree of physical activity is low. To protect their cardiovascular health and function a large proportion of the population must be motivated to abandon the sedentary lifestyle.

Ideas are needed. We know that people will improve if they take moderate rhythmic exercise regularly, say, five times each week, choosing an activity which requires the use of most of the large muscles of the body—for example, brisk walking or swimming. To be effective the exercise must be continued progressively longer week by week until it can be maintained for at least 30 minutes continuously. Other approaches may be effective and better suited to current patterns of daily life. Generally, the exercise taken should increase in integrity by small stages, each stage taking 8-10 weeks. This slow progression is particularly important for elderly or unfit people. The long term aim is, in general, to ensure that as many people as possible can at least walk a mile or more briskly on level ground.

The potential health gain from winning these changes in lifestyle is enormous.

SPORT FOR PEOPLE WITH DISABILITY

J C Chawla

Sport instills self discipline, a competitive spirit, and comradeship. Its value in promoting health, physical strength, endurance, social integration, and psychological wellbeing is of little doubt. It is not difficult to understand why sport is so important for the wellbeing of people with disability.

Some specific sporting activities have been developed for people with disability because of their inability to take part in ordinary sport. If due precautions are taken and adequate advice is given, however, most disabled people can participate in activities which are available to people without disability.

For many years disabled people have shown an interest in sport. Although opportunities for certain types of sport were available in the past, it was not until the passage of the Disabled Persons's Employment Act in 1944 that a major initiative was taken in the United Kingdom to provide facilities to enable disabled people to overcome handicaps that arose as a consequence of their disabilities. About the same time Sir Ludwig Guttman introduced sport as an essential part of the management of patients with spinal cord damage. He described the effects of sport on the rehabilitation of people with paraplegia and tetraplegia and stressed that sporting activities enabled them to overcome boredom in hospital and also promoted development of their physical and cardiorespiratory endurance.

The past five decades have seen an appreciable increase of interest in sport for disabled people not only in people with disability but also in the medical profession, sporting organisations, and the government. In 1978 the Sports Council stated that buildings to which they gave grant aid must provide facilities such as access for disabled people if they were to continue to qualify for aid.

Beneficial aspects of sport

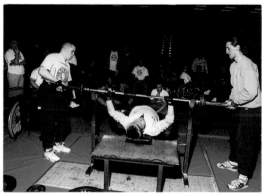

Weightlifting for people with a wide range of disabilities including visual or hearing impairment, paraplegia, or learning difficulties.

Treatment

A great many sporting activities that can be used for rehabilitation and recreation have become possible for disabled people. Sport is increasingly being used as treatment complementing the conventional methods of physiotherapy. It helps to develop strength, coordination, and endurance. Some sports develop selected groups of muscles—for example, weightlifting and archery help to strengthen the arm muscles of paraplegic patients, enabling them to gain independence in self care activities. Wheelchair sport such as basketball helps develop coordination as the disabled person has to propel the wheelchair and learn to pass, catch, and intercept the ball. Swimming is generally accepted as a valuable form of exercise and treatment. Over recent years it has become the most popular sport. When someone is immersed in water, mouth and nose above the surface while breathing, the buoyancy of the water allows limbs to move freely within that person's abilities.

Social benefits

Another important aspect of sport is the opportunities it provides for disabled people to establish social contacts. Disability that persists can cause deterioration of disabled people's attitudes towards themselves and result in self pity, disruption of self esteem, and social isolation. An adverse psychological reaction may be reinforced by the embarrassed attitude of the able bodied members of the community. Participation in sport can help newly physically disabled people to regain self esteem, promotes the development of positive mental attitudes, and helps them to come to terms with their disability and achieve social reintegration. Furthermore, disabled people with psychodepressive states have been seen to achieve resolution of this aspect of their disability by being able to take part in sport.

Sport and mental handicap

Mentally handicapped people appear to gain mental, social, spiritual, and physical benefits by involving themselves in the sport and leisure activities that have become available to them, but barriers to their participation still exist. It should be appreciated that mentally handicapped people may lack confidence and learn slowly. They may be reluctant to participate and may not be encouraged to do so by their parents or carers.

Sport for recreation

Over the years the realisation that recreational aspects of sport are important has led to the development of a wide range of outdoor activities, water sports, and indoor sports. Although integrated sport is desirable for all members of society, totally integrated facilities are not always possible. The sports that have become available to disabled people can be classified as:
- activities in which they may participate on equal terms with little or no modification (such as bowls, darts, archery, swimming, riding, table tennis);
- existing sport that has been modified (such as wheelchair basketball, darts, javelin throwing, weightlifting);
- sport that has been specially developed for disabled people (such as "roll ball" for visually handicapped people, Boccia ball).

Competitive sport

Increasing interest in sport has resulted in the development of competitive games. The competitive aspect of sport is important as it indicates a measure of attainment. As with sports for the able bodied, rules and regulations have been established. Different rules and classifications have been worked out for particular sports to enable disabled people to compete on equal terms. Classifications of disability are many and varied, some based on the cause of disability, others based on the parts of the body affected, such as arms, legs, heart.

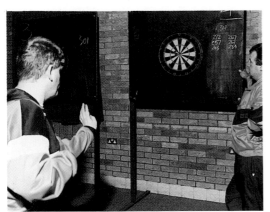
Sport in which able bodies and disabled people can integrate.

Disabilities recognised for international competition
- Paraplegia
- Amputation
- Locomotor disorders (les autres)
- Cerebral palsy
- Mental handicap
- Visual impairment
- Hearing impairment

Medical aspects

In general, disabled people consult their doctors before taking part in sporting activities and in some instances for a certificate of fitness, which may be required. Doctors need to assess their abilities and cardiorespiratory function and may be able to advise them if precautions are indicated. Some medical conditions may prevent people from participating in a particular sport. For example, people with low cardiorespiratory endurance, retinal detachment, or hernias are precluded from strenuous activities. A person with a healed cervical spine fracture or fused cervical spine should be advised against playing a contact sport such as rugby. Sports with risks of cuts and falls cannot be advocated for people with haemophilia.

Physical disabilities

The more severely disabled a person is the fewer are the sporting activities that he or she will be able to pursue. Some sporting activities such as angling, kite flying, and bird watching require very little physical effort, whereas others such as wheelchair basketball, riding,

---

Special sports needs of disabled people
- Specialist coaching
- Informed medical supervision
- Accessible facilities
- Information service

and sailing require coordination and strength in one or both arms. Sports such as hang gliding, canoeing, and surfing are not advisable for people with severe physical disability.

Physically disabled people undertake sports within the constraints of their mobility. Their doctors will therefore be concerned with preventing the usual complications of immobility and treating the injuries that may result from sporting activities. Some disabilities do not prevent participation but require precautions over and above the common ones. For example, people with paraplegia who are prone to spasms will need to use extra precautionary measures, such as body restraining straps, to prevent them from being thrown out of a wheelchair. Some people who have a combination of learning difficulties and physical disabilities require greater supervision than otherwise. Not all disabilities are static: some medical conditions such as multiple sclerosis may have a variable course and others such as muscular dystrophy are progressive. The sporting activity that is possible at one stage may not be so in the future. Medical reviews are necessary periodically to assess the individual's capacity to participate in sport.

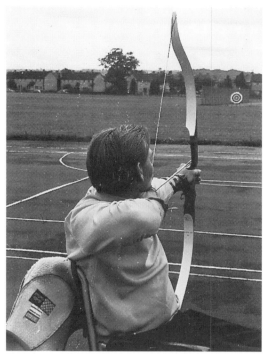

Archery helps strengthen arm muscles.

People with learning difficulties

Few reasons exist for restricting the participation of mentally handicapped people that cannot be overcome by developing a commonsense approach. Mentally handicapped patients who suffer from genetic disorders may have associated, potentially dangerous physical abnormalities such as congenital heart disease. In patients with Down's syndrome the potential instability of the atlantoaxial joint is of particular concern. Hyperextension or severe flexion of the cervical spine may produce severe neurological deficits or even death caused by compression of the lower brain stem and upper spinal cord. Opinions differ as to whether people with Down's syndrome should be allowed to take part in a contact sport. In the United States no restriction is placed on participation if there is no evidence of instability or the joint has been stabilised. In the United Kingdom, however, recommendations are that any activity likely to put undue strain on the cervical spine should not be encouraged. Although riding was not considered advisable for mentally handicapped people who have communication difficulties or behavioural disorders, over the past two decades they have been encouraged to ride.

People with acquired physical disabilities may have associated acquired mental handicap. They may have learning difficulties because of a not readily perceived cognitive deficit. Their inability to understand and retain information can result in frustration that may lead to behavioural disturbances.

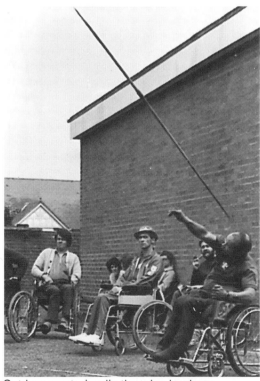

Outdoor sport—javelin throwing has been modified for disabled people.

Epilepsy

Epilepsy exposes the sufferers to many social disadvantages. They may be barred from driving or prevented from taking on certain employments. The term "epilepsy" includes different forms of seizures with a wide range of severity and control. Although patients with epilepsy but without physical disability or mental handicap are able to take part in any sport, restrictions are placed on their activities. Epileptic people who continue to have the occasional fit will pose a problem. The unpredictability of having fits, particularly if there is no aura, requires cautious advice. These patients are not allowed to participate in sub aqua diving. Activities such as canoeing or water skiing are not encouraged. The wearing of life jackets is an important addition to safety when sailing or rowing. The normal function of a life jacket is to turn the wearer on his or her back; a person who has suffered a seizure and is wearing a life jacket has a small risk of airway obstruction by the tongue falling back. An epileptic person should therefore be paired with a capable person who is familiar with the condition and knows what action to take if a seizure occurs.

Although caving may be possible when there is no ascent or descent by ladders, it should not be encouraged, because if rescue becomes necessary epilepsy will pose additional risks. Sports that are individualistic such as hang gliding should not be encouraged. People with epilepsy should be advised to take part in sporting activities where they do not endanger themselves or others and should be accompanied by someone who is familiar with their needs.

Visual impairment

People with visual impairment are generally fit unless there are other disabilities. Their movements, however, are not as free as those of people who have no visual impairment. The fear of falling or crashing against hard objects leads to stiffness of posture and movement and shuffling gait. Furthermore, acute loss of vision may be associated with an adverse psychological reaction. Sport and physical activity develop a sense of orientation in space and dynamic balance. As in other disabilities they help the visually impaired person to overcome frustrations and social isolation.

Visually impaired people are able to take part in many track and field events. Javelin, shot put, and club throwing have been practised by blind athletes for many years. They are able to take part in running, high jump, and long jump to name but a few. Blind people have a tendency to deviate from their course, which is usually corrected by a calling system. Similarly, in bowls the location of the jack is indicated by holding the arm of the bowler in that direction. Blind people are capable of swimming and their training does not materially differ from that of sighted people. Special sports such as roll ball have been developed for the blind.

The term blindness covers people with a great variety of visual deficits. Doctors and other professionals concerned with sport for the blind should appreciate that flashes of lights or blinking of stars may aggravate the visual impairment of partially sighted people.

Hearing impairment

Deaf people are capable of playing all sports that are open to people with normal hearing, though if the labyrinth is affected or acute deafness develops a deaf person may suffer from giddiness and disturbance of posture. Deaf people may be prevented from participating in sports that need good communication unless suitable arrangements are made.

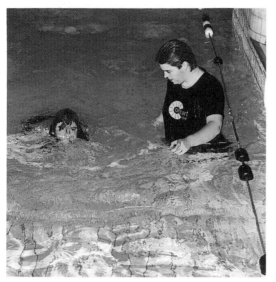

Swimming with attendant.

Assessment

Assessment of physically disabled people should also include assessment of orthotic and prosthetic devices, some of which may be hazardous in certain sports. It is usual to remove callipers and prosthetic legs when participating in water sports, as these may cause the wearer to sink. Buoyant artificial limbs are available to allow people who have had an amputation to take part in water sport. An artificial limb that is buoyant, however, can interfere with the function of a life jacket and prevent a person who is floating face down in water from turning over.

Disabled people seek information and advice from their medical advisers, who may not be fully aware of all aspects of the particular sporting activity being contemplated. If specific information is required, people should be directed towards a specialist who has a better understanding of what a particular sporting activity entails. In competitive sport the disabled person is examined by a doctor or member of the paramedical profession, usually a physiotherapist, both of whom are familiar with the classification systems. Attempts have been made over the years to improve classifications, basing them on people's abilities rather than disabilities.

Drugs

People with disability may be taking medication for control of a disease process or the symptoms, or both. Advising doctors should be aware of drugs that, if used, infringe the rules of the Sports Council. Self medication with certain products sold over the counter—for example, for a common cold, cough, pain, indigestion, etc—may contain banned substances. When in doubt, clarification should be sought from the appropriate governing body or the Sports Council.

Restricted drugs include:
- Sympathomimetic amines
- Central nervous system stimulants
- Antispasmodics
- Narcotic analgesics
- Non-steroidal anti-inflammatories
- Steroids
- Diuretics
- β Blockers
- Peptide hormones and their analogues

Conclusion

Useful sources of information:

British Wheelchair Sports Foundation, Guttman Sports Centre, Stoke Mandeville, Harvey Road, Aylesbury, Buckinghamshire HP21 9PP (0296 84848)

Disabled Living Foundation, 380-384 Harrow Road, London W9 2HU (071 289 6111)

Royal Association of Disability and Rehabilitation (RADAR), 25 Mortimer Street, London W1N 8AB (071 387 8033)

Royal National Institute for the Blind, 224 Great Portland Street, London W1N 6AA (071 388 1266)

Royal National Institute for the Deaf, 105 Gower Street, London WC1E 6AH (071 387 8033)

Royal Society for Mentally Handicapped Children and Adults (MENCAP), 117/123 Golden Lane, London EC1Y 0RT (071 454 0454)

Disability Action, 2 Annandale Avenue, Belfast BT7 (0232 491011)

Scottish Sports Association for the Disabled, 3 Martha Street, Glasgow G1 1GN (041 552 4807)

British Association of Sports and Medicine, The Reading Clinic, 10 Eldon Road, Reading RG1 4DH (0734 502 002)

Scottish Sports Council, Caledonia House, South Gyle, Edinburgh EH12 9DQ (031 317 7200)

Sports Council for Wales, Sophia Gardens, Cardiff CF1 9SW (0222 397571)

Local Disability Aid Centres—Addresses can be obtained from Disabled Living Centres Council (DLCC), 286 Camden Road, London N7 0BJ (071 700 1707)

Local Leisure Centres

Doctors should be concerned not only with identifying risk factors, the ability of individual people, and potential hazards but also with the benefits that sport can offer to disabled people. Doctors active in sport for disabled people must familiarise themselves with the requirements of particular sports, the consequences of disabilities, and the abilities of the disabled people. With improved equipment and training programmes a disabled person is able to achieve far more than might be expected. The value of sport, and the fact that disabled people are not a homogeneous group having been recognised, a close dialogue between the medical profession, sports scientists, coaches, sporting authorities, and disabled people themselves is necessary to ensure that people with disability can achieve the maximum within their capacity in the sporting activities of their choice.

FITNESS FOR OLDER PEOPLE

Archie Young, Susie Dinan

Benefits

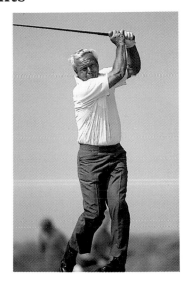

Throughout life the health benefits of regular, vigorous, physical activity far outweigh the hazards. Moreover, the hazards can be reduced by education and guidance of participants.

Prevention of disease

Regular exercise helps prevent conditions important in old age, notably osteoporosis, non-insulin dependent diabetes mellitus, hypertension, ischaemic heart disease, and probably stroke.

Prevention of disability

Not only does regular exercise have important effects in preventing disease but its effects in preserving function are also important. Appropriate physical training improves the functional abilities of people with disabling symptoms of intermittent claudication, angina pectoris, heart failure, asthma, and chronic bronchitis. Even frail older patients with multiple disabilities may also derive functional benefits from graded physical training.

Even healthy older people lose strength (the ability to exert force) at some 1-2% a year and power (force×speed) at some 3-4% a year. In addition, many older people have further problems because of chronic disease. The resulting weakness has important functional consequences for the performance of everyday activities. A similar argument applies for endurance capacity.

Regular exercise increases strength, endurance, and flexibility. In percentage terms, the improvements seen in older people are similar to those in younger people. For example, in a recent study in our laboratory, women aged 75 to 93 training three times a week for 12 weeks increased their strength by 24-30%, equivalent to a "rejuvenation" of strength by 16-20 years.

Prevention of immobility

For severely disabled people, immobility itself brings substantial hazards. For them just movement itself, even in the absence of a training effect, is crucial in preventing, for example, faecal impaction (and incontinence), deep vein thrombosis (and pulmonary embolism), and gravitational oedema (and skin ulceration).

Prevention of isolation

In addition to its physiological effects, recreational exercise offers important opportunities for socialisation. It also permits the emotional benefits of socially acceptable touching, unconnected with dependence and the need for personal care, a rarity for many long-bereaved, older people.

Preventive effects of exercise

Disease, such as:
- Osteoporosis
- Non-insulin dependent diabetes
- Hypertension
- Ischaemic heart disease
- Stroke

Disability caused by:
- Intermittent claudication
- Angina pectoris
- Heart failure
- Asthma
- Chronic bronchitis

Immobility, which can cause:
- Faecal impaction
- Incontinence
- Deep vein thrombosis
- Pulmonary embolism
- Gravitational oedema
- Skin ulceration

Isolation, which can cause:
- Loneliness
- Depression

Providing guidance and opportunity

Any exercise programme to improve general fitness should include activities that develop strength, endurance, flexibility, and coordination in a progressive, balanced, and enjoyable way. All major muscle groups should be used in exercises that train through a full range of movement. An exercise programme for older people must also aim to load the bones, target postural and pelvic floor muscles, and develop body awareness and balance skills. A combination of recreational brisk walking and swimming will meet most of these criteria for most people. Many, however, will also welcome the opportunity to participate in an exercise group.

Exercise classes

This chapter offers guidance to health professionals on aspects to consider when they assess an exercise class to which they might refer patients, or when they seek specialist training to enable them to conduct such sessions safely and successfully.

All sessions should start and finish gradually. The warm up loosens joints, rehearses skills, warms and stretches muscles, and gradually increases demand on heart and lungs. The "warm down" incorporates held stretches and relaxation but consists principally of slow rhythmic exercises to preserve venous return as muscle and skin vasodilation gradually return to resting levels.

Many of the activities should be closely related to lifestyle and to maintaining independence. Techniques of lifting, walking, and transferring (moving from sitting to standing, standing to lying, etc) should be specifically taught and discussed. Information about the specific benefits of particular exercises is greatly appreciated—for example, increasing shoulder mobility for doing up zips, building up stamina for "energy" and less breathlessness during exertion, or strengthening quadriceps, handgrip, and biceps for lifting holiday suitcases.

But, above all, fitness must be fun. Important factors can be the use of appropriate music and opportunities for socialising (but beware of making agist assumptions about what is appropriate).

Programming

The aim is a long term commitment to a mixture of activities. The combinations should be tailored to individual fitness levels, tastes, and interests and might include walking, swimming, cycling, exercise to music, weight training, circuit training, step training, dancing, tai chi, tennis, bowls, etc. A home exercise programme can usefully complement the organised sessions. Provision must be made for a wide range of initial levels of habitual physical activity and a variety of disabilities.

Programmes should provide some sessions exclusive to older people and others integrated with other age groups for selected activities. Opportunities to socialise should be scheduled at all activities. Year round programming is essential. Off peak timing improves use of resources but must not exclude the many older people still in employment. Qualified teachers should be paid, but concessionary charges and discretionary financial assistance for participants should be considered.

Participants must be involved in planning, selecting, and evaluating the programme. The setting should be convenient for older people in respect of public transport, parking, access, ambience, ventilation, lighting, refreshments, changing and toilet facilities, and floor surfaces and thought should also be given to those with a disability (for example, by providing stair rails, large print notices, and wheelchair access). Promotional material should feature appropriate older role models.

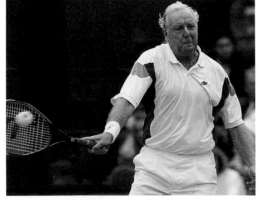

A player in the 45 and over tournament at Wimbledon.

Safety

Injury prevention is a high priority. Even stiffness and minor overuse injuries reduce enjoyment and adherence to a programme, and can often be avoided. An adequate warm up, the selection of safe exercises and movement patterns, and regular monitoring of body alignment and exercise intensity are important. Precise, audible teaching instructions and visible, skilled demonstrations are essential. Good class management and observation are needed to ensure safety in "seniors'" fitness sessions. These issues are all taught in specialist courses for those training to run fitness for seniors sessions. Competence to run such sessions (see "Qualifications") implies both theoretical knowledge and practical experience in selecting safe and appropriate exercises for people with particular types of medical problem—for example, those who are unsteady, are breathless, have angina, or are chairbound. It also implies the ability to recognise significant new symptoms during exercise.

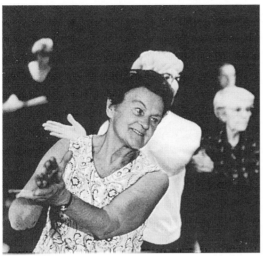
The use of appropriate music can make exercise more fun.

Opinion is divided over use of informed consent and the use of medical release forms. Nevertheless, exercise teachers will usually instruct older people to consult their doctor before embarking on a programme of exercise to which they are unaccustomed. The doctor has two responsibilities. Firstly, to identify the disorders that are present and to ensure that they will be accurately communicated to the exercise teacher. Secondly, to educate the potential exerciser in the early recognition of symptoms that might indicate that their exercise programme is in some way unsuitable for them and their particular chronic disorders. Thus, for example, the patient with osteoarthritic knees should be taught to recognise and respect an increase in pain, stiffness, or swelling. The patient with a history of mild, controlled, heart failure should be taught that shortness of breath during exercise is normal but that a decrease in the level of exercise required to provoke it is abnormal.

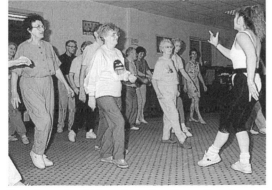
Exercises should be safe and well monitored.

Qualifications

In many respects an older person is like an athlete; both often perform near their limits. The coaching skills required to ensure both optimum performance and safety are important and specialised. There is a recognised qualification developed and awarded by London Central YMCA (validated by the Royal Society of Arts, and approved by the Sports Council), which is held by fitness teachers who have been trained to work with people aged 50 and over. To be eligible for the specialist courses leading to this qualification, the exercise teacher must already hold an appropriate certificate from the Royal Society of Arts (in exercise to music) or from the London Central YMCA or the Physical Education Association (in fitness training) and have at least six months' teaching experience. Health professionals can also train for the 50 plus qualification via the London Central YMCA's access or in service courses. In addition, especially for those working with older people with disabilities, "Extend" offers instruction and certification.

Conclusion

> The physical and psychological benefits of exercise in older people are considerable

Health professionals are well placed to endorse the "use it or lose it" message and give the advice, encouragement, or even "permission" that older people often need to begin or to return to physical recreation. In partnership with trained exercise teachers and other community agencies they can make a major contribution to the health (and happiness) of the nation.

Useful contacts

Training

Royal Society of Arts (RSA) Examinations Board, Progress House, Westwood Way, Coventry CV4 8HS (0203 470033)

Extend, 22 Maltings Drive, Wheathamstead, Herts AL4 8QJ (0582) 832760)

Agencies

Sports Council, 16 Upper Woburn Place, London WC1H 0QP (071 388 1277)

Sports Council for Wales, Welsh Institute of Sport, Sophia Gardens, Cardiff CF1 9SW (0222 397571)

Age Concern England, (Age Well) (Age Resource), Astral House, 1268 London Road, Norbury, London SW16 4ER (081 679 8000)

Age Concern Wales, 4th Floor, 1 Cathedral Road, Cardiff CF1 9SD (0222 371566)

Association of Retired Persons, Greencourt House, Frances Street, London SW1P 1D2 (071 895 8800)

Physical Education Association of Great Britain, Ling House, 5 Western Court, Bromley Street, Digbeth, Birmingham B9 4AN (021 753 0909)

The Exercise Association of England, Unit 4, Angel Gate, 326 City Road, London EC1V 2PT (071 278 0811)

London Central YMCA (Training and Development), 112 Great Russell Street, London WC1B 3NQ (071 580 2989).
(Also regional offices throughout the UK)

Scottish Sports Council, Caledonia House, South Gyle, Edinburgh EH12 9DQ (031 317 7200)

Sports Council for Northern Ireland, House of Sport, Upper Malone Road, Belfast BT9 5LA (0232 381222)

Age Concern Scotland, 54a Fountainbridge, Edinburgh EH3 9PT (031 228 5656)

Age Concern Northern Ireland, 3 Lower Crescent, Belfast BT7 1NR (0232 245729)

Help the Aged (Sportage), St James's Walk, London EC1R 0BE

Ramblers Association, 1/5 Wandsworth Road, London SW8 2XX (071 582 6878)

Multi-purpose fitness equipment suitable for older people
Davies, The Sports People (Nottingham Rehabilitation Equipment), 1 Ludlow Hill Road, West Bridgford, Nottingham NG2 6HD (0602 452345)

The photograph of the golfer is reproduced with permission from Colorsport, and that of the Wimbledon veteran by Allsport. The two photographs of exercise classes are reproduced by permission of London Central YMCA.

FEMALE ATHLETES

Roslyn Carbon

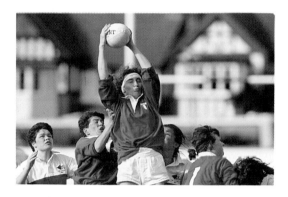

Female athletes now compete in virtually all the main sporting arenas of the world in which the physical differences between the sexes are largely irrelevant because women only compete against men in certain technique events. Social and historical influences remain the most important factors determining the participation and success of female athletes. A Chinese women, Zhang Chan, scored a perfect 200 in the skeet (clay pigeon) shooting competition to take the gold medal and world record at the Barcelona Olympics, but will be unable to defend her title when the event is an all male contest in Atlanta in 1996.

Physical differences between the sexes

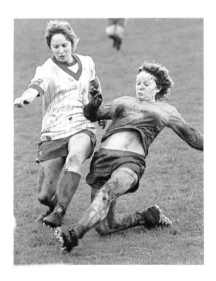

Women are, on average, 10% smaller than men in most physical variables including cardiac size, blood volume, and haemoglobin concentration. However, they carry twice the body fat of men. The net result is a lower total aerobic capacity of some 40%. Yet if maximal oxygen uptake is expressed as a percentage of lean body weight the difference is less than 10%. Women are capable of appreciable improvements in muscle strength without demonstrable increases in muscle bulk in the early stages of weight training as a result of improved neuromuscular recruitment. In general, however, muscle strength is equivalent in both sexes for the same cross sectional area of muscle.

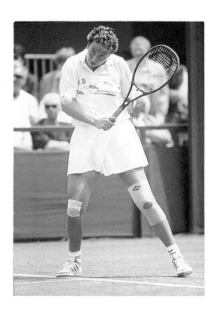

The effect of power and aerobic training results in physical adaptation whereby the differences between male and female trained athletes are far less than those between sedentary men and women. Women excel in ultra-endurance events and currently hold most of the world records in long distance swimming. The physiology of this supremacy is not well understood but may relate to improved fat metabolism, local muscle endurance at low workloads, tolerance of temperature extremes, and greater bouyancy in water.

As women have historically been prohibited from playing body contact sports they do not suffer much of the major trauma experienced by sportsmen. Early statistics, especially military data on new recruits, indicated that women were more prone to injuries than men, but recent research has shown this to be more a product of the poor initial fitness of the women in these programmes. Most injuries are more sport specific than sex specific, although data from professional sport in the United States indicate a possibly higher level of severe intra-articular knee injuries in women basketball players.

Gender verification

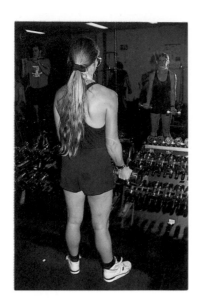

Because of the obvious advantages in strength and size of men over women it has long been accepted that the two sexes should compete in separate competitions. During the 1960s, when women began hard physical training, and perhaps because of the advent of misuse of anabolic steroids, there were increasing concerns regarding the sexuality of some female athletes. It was decided by the major sporting organisations that all women should undergo "gender verification" to prove their feminity.

The first attempt at sex testing by the International Amateur Athletic Federation in 1966 involved the parade of naked female athletes before a panel of male doctors. Fortunately this was immediately replaced by the International Olympic Committee with the buccal smear test for the Barr body (X chromatin). At the Barcelona Games in 1992 the Barr test was replaced by the polymerase chain reaction (PCR) test, which detects the presence of the Y chromosome. The buccal smear is minimally invasive, is inoffensive, and gives rapid results. It does not, however, detect women abnormally virilised by such conditions as congenital adrenal hyperplasia, but it does show the chromosomal abnormality (XY) of phenotypic women with testicular feminisation. The latter undergo physical examination to assess their phenotype and are allowed to compete in Olympic competition.

There is a strong lobby group within the scientific and medical community to stop gender screening. Certainly, because of the flaws of the buccal screening procedure, any sporting organisation that intends to undertake gender verification must have the appropriate medical and administrative expertise.

Reproductive function and exercise

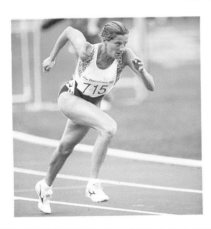

Though the genitalia of men risk greater trauma in sporting contests, the reproductive physiology of the female athlete appears most susceptible to the stresses of competition and hard training.

Menstruation itself has long ceased to represent any bar to sport or exercise, and there is no convincing evidence that athletic ability is consistently altered by the phases of the cycle. For women with dysmenorrhoea or premenstrual symptoms it is reasonable to offer treatment with monophasic oral contraceptives or progestagens that alter the menstrual cycle or delay bleeding. Alternatively, simple analgesia or non-steroidal anti-inflammatory drugs can be used to control pain. Care should be taken not to give proscribed drugs such as diuretics to competitive athletes.

Oligomenorrhoea and amenorrhoea

Some athletic women experience altered menstrual cycles, but this is rarely if ever a result of their sporting activity alone. These athletes are usually thin young runners, dancers, or gymnasts who have inadequate diets for their exercise level. So called "athletic amenorrhoea" is a form of hypothalamic dysfunction in which the pulsatile release of gonadotrophin releasing hormone is altered, with a resultant decrease in secretion of pituitary gonadotrophins and subsequent secondary ovarian failure. Primary amenorrhoea—delayed menarche—is also common in some groups of sportswomen including dancers, but is also probably related to self selection of these athletes.

Rather than representing an on/off mechanism, the menstrual change is a gradual depression of the hypothalamic-pituitary-ovarian axis along a continuum, which may start with shortening of the luteal phase, leading to prolonged anovulatory cycles and thence to established amenorrhoea. The exact cause of this form of amenorrhoea remains unknown but may be related to feedback mechanisms from increased secretion of endorphin or cortisol, or both, in response to physical and emotional stress levels. Altered gonadotrophin concentrations are not unique to female athletes as male marathon runners have also been reported to have low luteinising hormone concentrations and sperm counts.

Relevant physical examination in athletes with amenorrhoea

- Height, weight, sum of skinfolds, body mass index
- Pulse rate and body temperature (may be low in anorexia nervosa)
- "Lanugo" hair and parotid swelling (evidence of eating disorder)
- Galactorrhoea on gentle nipple compression (evidence of hyperprolactinaemia)
- Hirsutism, acne, clitoromegaly (signs of virilisation)
- Pulse rate, eye signs, tremor (signs of thyroid disease)
- Perineal examination, especially in primary amenorrhoea
- Pelvic examination for anatomical abnormalities
- Cervical smear (if indicated) may give cellular evidence of gonadal steroid inadequacy

Athletic amenorrhoea can be viewed as a (mal)adaptation that is also associated with high incidence of injury and is part of a global "overstressing" or overtraining in the individual. To reduce the incidence of primary and secondary amenorrhoea, sporting associations should discourage strong pressures on athletes to achieve waif-like stature with delayed maturation while competing in arduous sporting programmes.

Differential diagnosis of athletic amenorrhoea

- Eating disorder
- Pregnancy
- Hyperprolactinaemia
- Primary ovarian failure
- Virilisation syndromes including misuse of anabolic steroids
- Polycystic ovarian disease
- Thyroid disease
- Genetic disorders ⎫ (primary
- Anatomical abnormalities ⎬ amenorrhoea)

Diagnosis of amenorrhoea

Athletes should always be thoroughly assessed to diagnose and treat other possible causes of amenorrhoea. Athletic amenorrhoea is characterised by low follicle stimulating hormone (FSH), luteinising hormone (LH), oestrogen E2), and progesterone concentrations. Physical examination (despite often disclosing low body fat) is normal, as are thyroid function and serum prolactin and androgen concentrations.

Relevant investigations in athletes with amenorrhoea

- Serum concentrations of:

    oestradiol
    progesterone
    follicle stimulating hormone
    luteinising hormone
    prolactin
    testosterone, dehydroepiandrosterone

- Thyroid function tests

(NB All blood tests must be taken after at least 24 hours rest from activity)

- Pelvic ultrasonography (preferable to full pelvic examination in young athletes). Note that cystic ovaries may be non-specific

- Cranial computed tomography or magnetic resonance imaging scan for pituitary tumour (if prolactin concentration is raised)

- Bone density—for example, dual energy *x* ray absorptiometry (DEXA)

Factors associated with menstrual changes in athletes

Menstrual regularity	*Menstrual irregularity*
Maturity of reproductive axis	Youth
Established ovulatory cycles	Nulliparity
Advanced gynaecological age	Decreased bodyweight
Parity	Decreased body fat
Increased bodyweight	Low energy diet
Increased body fat	High volume, high intensity exercise
Gradual increase in activity	Rapid increase in exercise workload
Low intensity exercise	Psychological stress

Bone mineral density

Despite their high levels of exercise, women with athletic amenorrhoea are likely to have decreased trabecular bone density as a result of low gonadal steroid concentrations. Cortical bone density, which is increased by weightbearing physical activity, remains normal. Several studies have reported a higher rate of stress fracture in athletes with amenorrhoea. This may represent part of the overall increase in injury or be a result of low bone mass itself. However, these fractures occur mostly in weightbearing cortical bone and not in areas of measured osteopenia, and as yet the relation between amenorrhoea, stress fractures, and bone mineral density remains unexplained.

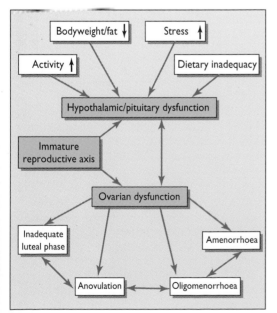

Factors affecting menstrual change in athletes.

It is important to remember that physical activity itself is a potent stimulator of bone deposition and should be encouraged in young girls to increase peak bone mass and in older women to delay bone loss.

Female athletes

Management

Athletic amenorrhoea is itself almost invariably reversible when the stresses responsible for its development are eliminated. Menses and fertility are restored in all but a very small proportion of women who have never developed a normal reproductive axis. Longitudinal research, however, has shown that the shortfall in bone density from prolonged amenorrhoea may not be restored after resumption of menses. As in postmenopausal women most of the bone loss occurs early in the hypo-oestrogenic state and for this reason athletic amenorrhoea should not be ignored as being a benign condition.

The most appropriate management is attention to the factors responsible for the amenorrhoea. Athletes should be advised to eat a well balanced diet supplying sufficient energy to match their energy expenditure and should be encouraged to gain weight. Training should be decreased, initially by 10-20%. In practice many top level athletes may not heed such advice. Progestagens alone or oestrogen and progestagen combinations such as postmenopausal preparations, or the contraceptive pill may be used—especially if there is concern regarding bone mass.

Exercise and pregnancy

Previous concerns of the medical profession about the childbearing capacities of athletic women have not been borne out. Similarly, concerns regarding the safety of exercise by pregnant women have largely been overstated. A large body of research over the past two decades has confirmed that maternal exercise is well tolerated by the fetus at least up to 70% of maximum exercise. Many of the physiological changes in early pregnancy, such as increased blood volume and hyperventilation with alkalosis, are in fact advantageous to maternal exercise. Women have competed in major sporting events such as Wimbledon while pregnant and even completed marathons in the third trimester. There are no published reports of fetal compromise or adverse outcome of pregnancy as a result of maternal exercise and, with few exceptions, regular exercise should be viewed as a healthy part of normal pregnancy.

Clearly, medical problems occur within pregnancy that present relative or absolute contraindications to exercise. Guidelines offered by various medical bodies centre on the following three major topics of concern.

Trauma

The fetus is well protected within the pelvis and later by the layers of the abdominal wall and uterus with the amniotic fluid. However, largely for medicolegal reasons, most sporting bodies bar pregnant women from participating beyond the second trimester.

Hyperthermia and dehydration

Animal studies and retrospective data in women have indicated that maternal hyperthermia is a risk factor for neural tube defects. The prolonged fever (>39°C for three days) cited in these reports, however, does not equate with the mild temperature changes experienced during most exercise. Sensible guidelines would include exercising during the cool period of the day and ensuring adequate hydration.

Placental perfusion

Animal studies indicating that maternal exercise diverts blood flow from the uterus to working muscle raised concern regarding perfusion of the fetus. Cardiotocography studies indicate, however, that the fetus accommodates such blood flow changes well, responding with moderate and temporary tachycardia. Changes are less evident if the mother is aerobically trained, and further haemodynamic compensation includes preferential shunting of blood to the placenta and increased oxygen transfer in response to the high oxygen affinity of fetal haemoglobin.

> Committed athletes need emphatic antenatal care to combine healthy pregnancy with their training aspirations.

Athletic mothers

The concept that women suffer an inevitable decline in sporting prowess after motherhood is no longer tenable. Indeed, many sporting authorities consider childbearing an asset to performance, though whether the beneficial long term effects are physical or psychological is not known.

Conclusion

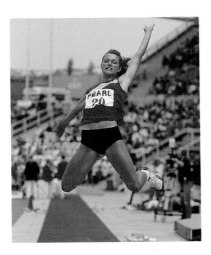

The vast majority of female athletes are healthy fertile women and this is evidenced by the large number of athletes who succeed into motherhood. There is no scientific evidence that any form of physical exercise is uniquely harmful to women. Doctors should play a prominent role in promoting the health benefits of exercise for women and ensuring the best management for any health or injury problems of female athletes.

The photographs of women's rugby and the long jumper were taken by Supersport Photographs, that of women's football by John Walmsley, those of the woman tennis player and the runner by Professional Sport, and that of the woman weightlifter (© the Sports Council) by Richard J Sowersby.

TEMPERATURE AND PERFORMANCE

Evan L Lloyd

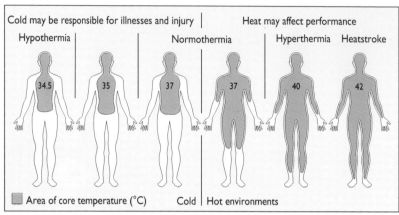

Cold may be responsible for illnesses and injury | Heat may affect performance

Hypothermia | Normothermia | Hyperthermia | Heatstroke

34.5 | 35 | 37 | 37 | 40 | 42

■ Area of core temperature (°C) Cold | Hot environments

Rough relation of core temperatures and shell sizes. (Note the arbitrary temperature definition of hypothermia (<35°C) and the range of shell sizes in normothermia.)

The rate of dry heat loss (convection and conduction) depends on the temperature difference between the skin and the environment. The rate of evaporative heat loss (surface evaporation and through breathing) depends on the ambient humidity. Air movement (air over the body or the body through the air) increases both types of heat loss.

COLD

Hypothermia

> ### Types of hypothermia
>
> *Immersion*—Very severe cold stress occurs, for example, in a sailor or canoeist who capsizes
>
> *Exhaustion*—Less severe cold stress, most frequently a combination of wind and wet with moderately low temperatures. Usually found in mountaineers or hill walkers but also in cross country skiers, runners, cyclists, and others who participate in endurance events
>
> *Urban*—Cold is relatively mild but prolonged. Most common in elderly people or those with malnutrition but not in normal sport

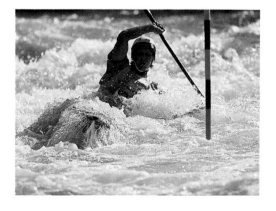

When estimating the severity of cold stress—that is, the rate of heat loss—wind and wet are as important as temperature. A body is in fact losing more heat at +10°C in a 20 mph wind than at −10°C in still air.

Hypothermia will develop if the rate of heat loss from the body exceeds the rate at which the body is producing heat. Suitable conditions may occur in many sports and at any time of year. There are three physiologically distinct types of hypothermia, and inappropriate treatment may cause death.

Though drowning is the commonest cause of death in water, in cold water hypothermia may predispose to and accompany drowning.

Diagnosis

Firstly, suspect the possibility of hypothermia. The earliest symptom is usually a change in behaviour (but similar symptoms occur in hyperthermia, exhaustion, and hypoglycaemia). This is followed by incoordination, staggering, dysarthria, a progressive clouding and loss of consciousness, and slowing of heart and respiration with death as the final outcome. Accurate diagnosis can be made only by measuring the core temperature, usually rectally, but the necessary low reading thermometer is unlikely to be available where casualties occur. For practical purposes a casualty should be treated as a "cold casualty" if the body feels "as cold as marble," particularly if the armpit is profoundly cold.

Management before admission to hospital

With all three types of hypothermia, prevent further heat loss by removing the casualty from the cold environment. Movement must be gentle to avoid triggering a cardiac arrest, but in a severe environment such as cold water the priority is to get the person out of the cold. Until the casualty is indoors, wet clothes should not be removed, but layers of insulating material should be put on top of the clothing and covered with a layer that is water and wind proof. The head must be included. Space blankets are often recommended but are no more effective than a similar thickness of very much cheaper polythene. If available, airway warming (the inhalation of warmed moist air) should be used. This treatment is of particular value in exhaustion hypothermia where it will prevent the sometimes fatal cardiovascular collapse that may occur during rewarming. Moderate surface warmth is dangerous in exhaustion hypothermia. Casualties with hypothermia should be taken to hospital for rewarming with intensive care monitoring. With urban hypothermia no additional heat, either surface or central, should be supplied before admission to hospital as this will precipitate fatal pulmonary or cerebral oedema or both, by reversing fluid shifts between compartments. These shifts can be monitored and controlled in intensive care.

Resuscitation after hypothermia

Respiratory obstruction should be cleared and, if necessary, expired air ventilation started using the same criteria and rate as in normothermia. Cardiopulmonary resuscitation, at the same rate as in normothermia, should be started if indicated.

Casualties totally submerged in very cold water, especially those who are young, have been known to recover even after submersion of up to one hour. Resuscitation must start immediately on rescue.

Frostbite

Frostbite is a localised lesion caused by freezing. It preferentially affects the periphery—feet, hands, ears, nose, and cheeks—though the cornea has been affected in downhill skiers and speed skaters not protected by goggles. Penile freezing can occur during skiing or running in tight or inadequate clothing or from direct contact with a metal zip. Anything that restricts the circulation, such as tight training shoes, increases the risk, as does dehydration, excess tiredness, and altitude.

In *frostnip* the exposed skin, which has been painful, blanches and loses sensation but remains pliable. The part should be warmed by placing it in the armpit or under clothing. The part tingles, becomes hyperaemic, and within a few minutes, sensation is restored and normal activity can be resumed.

In *frostbite* the tissues are hard, insensitive, and white or mottled. No attempt should be made to thaw frostbite if there is any chance of the part becoming refrozen because freeze-thaw-refreeze causes more damage than continuous freezing. It is safer to walk on frozen feet even for 72 hours.

Treatment—Rewarming is ideally done in a hot (40°C) whirlpool bath, with gradual spontaneous rewarming as second best. Beating, rubbing with snow, or rewarming with excessive heat produce disastrous loss of tissue. Because damage from frostbite is usually more superficial than first suspected, debridement or amputation should be delayed for up to 90 days till mummification and demarcation are complete. After recovery the sufferer can return to full activity limited only by any tissue loss.

Trench foot

This develops over a fairly long period when the legs are exposed to cold (above freezing) or wet, or both—for example, prolonged walking in boggy ground or sweating in impervious boots. As in frostbite, damage is more likely if there is fatigue, dehydration, immobility, and tight footwear. The feet are initially cold and numb, giving the sensation of "walking on cotton wool" and the combination with joint stiffness causes the victim to walk with legs apart to maintain balance. When first seen the feet are cold, swollen, and blotchy pink-purple or blanched.

Treatment—Remove the person from the hostile environment and allow the part to rewarm spontaneously. After rewarming, feet become hyperaemic, hot, and red with paraesthesia or pain which may be severe (like electric shocks) especially on weight bearing. This may last for weeks. Severe cases cause bleeding into the skin, ulceration, and blisters and may progress to gangrene.

Because of the nerve and other damage, there is likely to be persistent, or permanent, hypersensitivity to cold as well as anaesthesia or hyperaesthesia and problems with the bony structure of the feet.

Indications for starting cardiopulmonary resuscitation in hypothermia

(1) No carotid pulse is detectable for at least one minute

OR

Cardiac arrest is observed—that is, a pulse disappears—or there is a reasonable chance that cardiac arrest occurred within the previous two hours

AND

(2) There is a reasonable expectation that effective cardiopulmonary resuscitation can be continued, with only brief periods of interruption for movement, until the casualty can be transported to hospital, where full advanced life support can be provided

Local effects of cold

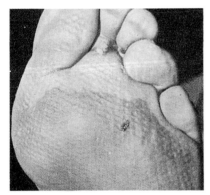

Cold rigid foot without sensation or digital motion. Note marks of sock texture. Extensive clear blisters developed, which became black when dry but finally sloughed off leaving normal function and anatomy. (Blood filled blisters, however, are a bad sign.)

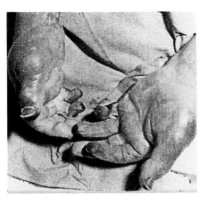

Hands less than 24 hours after frostbite thawed by using excess heat (boiling water in this case). Hands are cyanotic, painful, and foul smelling and there are no blebs. Resulted in spontaneous amputation at the metacarpophalangeal junction at six weeks.

Other effects of cold

Other effects of cold exposure

Muscular
    Shivering
    Incapacity in very cold water

Cardiovascular
    Angina on decreased exertion
    Rise in blood pressure—increases risk of:
        Stroke
        Myocardial infarction
        Heart failure

Respiratory
    Exercise/asthma—worse in cold
    Rhinorrhoea on return to warm room
    Increased susceptibility to upper respiratory infection
    Uncontrollable hyperventilation in sudden severe cold—even if fully
        submerged
    Loss of consciousness
    Disabled by tetany

Nervous system
    Loss of manual dexterity and sensitivity
    Coordination impaired
    Visual acuity and alertness reduced
    Reflexes slowed
    Increased mistakes
    Visual and auditory sensory input misinterpreted
    Hallucinations

Other
    Increased risk of "bends"
    Allergy—possible anaphylactic shock

Muscle injury

Muscle and tendon tears occur when a person is cold, and inactive muscles are cold even in warm weather.

Prevention—Stretching, and an active and adequate warm up (till the limbs feel "glowing warm" and there is a slight feeling of breathlessness) are the most effective means for reducing the risk of injury and enhancing performance. The little evidence there is suggests that massage, even skilled massage for 30 minutes, is mainly of psychological benefit and a hot shower is useless in place of a warm up.

Sudden exposure to cold may result in death before there is any drop in core temperature. In cold water this may be secondary to an incapacity that leads to drowning. In very cold water even Olympic class swimmers become incapacitated, but the effects are reduced if a person is acclimatised to cold immersion by habituation training.

Very cold water in the ears or nose may cause instantaneous cardiac and respiratory arrest. Cold in the ears may also lead to disorientation, which can cause submerged people, such as capsized canoeists, to swim downwards instead of towards the surface.

HEAT

Heatstroke

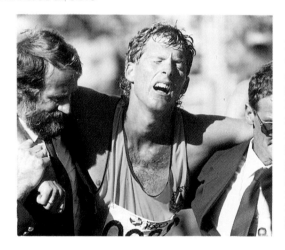

Heatstroke develops when the body is unable to get rid of the excess heat being produced. There will be a varying combination of high environmental temperature, high humidity, lack of wind, vigorous activity, heat retaining clothing, and dehydration. Early symptoms include excessive sweating, headache, nausea, dizziness, hyperventilation, and disturbance of consciousness. Consciousness may be lost or clouded and there may be hallucinations. There may be muscle twitching or convulsions and loss of control of the body sphincters. In severe cases there may be deep coma with pinpoint pupils. They may be in shock with tachycardia. Tachypnoea is often present and breathing may be difficult and vomit inhaled. The patient feels warm or hot and has a high core temperature (rectal usually >41°C). Sweating may or may not be present. Diagnosis depends on a high index of suspicion.

Treatment of heatstroke

(1) Lie the patient flat and raise the legs

(2) Cool by removing clothing within modesty, spraying with warm or tepid water, and fanning with warm air

Do NOT use ice baths, ice packs, cold sponging, or blowing cold air. This may kill the patient because the cold stimulus causes vasoconstriction, thus reducing heat loss, and triggers shivering, thus increasing heat production

(3) Rehydrate with sodium rich fluid like 0·9% saline. Several litres may be required to restore or maintain blood pressure. Intravenous bicarbonate will be needed to counteract the metabolic acidosis but this is best done in hospital by measuring acid/base status. Hydrocortisone (repeated doses of 100 mg intravenously) may be necessary if the blood pressure is falling

(4) Transer to the intensive care unit in a hospital

Management

Without correct treatment a heatstroke victim is in great danger of developing irreversible damage in the brain, kidneys, liver, and adrenal glands, or of death. Disseminated intravascular coagulation may occur. Treatment should be started as early as possible. Unnecessary cooling is much safer than waiting for a definite diagnosis.

Local effects of heat

Treatment of sunburn
Avoid further exposure
Mild sunburn   Cool soak—tap water
Emollients
Aspirin and other non-steroidal anti-inflammatory drugs
Topical steroids
Severe sunburn *(blistering)*
As for mild sunburn plus:
Prednisolone oral 60 mg/day, tapering in one week
Protect bullae if intact
Admit to hospital

Sunburn

Unprotected exposure to sun causes sunburn and depresses immune responses in the skin leading to recurrent herpes labialis—for example in skiers. It also increases the risk of skin cancer—basal and squamous cell carcinomas on exposed areas and melanomas anywhere on the body. The risks are increased by altitude, by reflective surfaces (such as fresh ice, snow, water (especially morning and evening), sand, metal, concrete, and by wind ("windburn" is exacerbated sunburn). Sunburn can occur unexpectedly during cloudy weather.

Prevention is by using clothing, and sunscreens according to skin type. Sunscreens should protect against UVA and UVB and be water resistant. Unfortunately treatment for sunburn may be necessary.

Other effects of heat

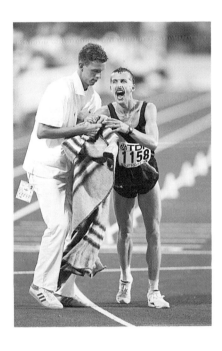

Dehydration, loss of performance, collapse

In high environmental temperatures, 60% of cardiac output may pass through the skin for cooling and sweat production, and unacclimatised people will therefore perform less well in heat. Loss of fluid of 1% of body weight (600-800 ml) by sweating will lead to reduced performance. To prevent dehydration people should drink at least an extra cupful of water every hour (1½-2 litres a day) and be weighed three times a day because rapid weight loss in the heat means water loss not fat loss. People losing weight should therefore drink more—possibly even 10 litres—to maintain body weight. Urine should be plentiful and light coloured. Urine that is dark, strong smelling, or of reduced volume means the person has a large fluid deficit.

Salt depletion from sweating causes tiredness, irritability, giddiness, fainting, cramps, and loss of performance. During the first 10 days in the heat additional salt should be taken as salt tablets or dilute (0·1%) solution. A normal diet should provide enough other electrolytes.

Hyperventilation is usually an indication of possible heatstroke. Occasionally a person who has a reduced ability to sweat, increases heat loss by tachypnoea and by panting, producing uncompensated respiratory alkalosis with unconsciousness and tetanic spasm. This occurs after a competitor has appeared normal at the end of the event, and it will resolve completely with simple rest. In heatstroke there is unlikely to be tetanic spasm, but hyperventilation in an athlete should lead to a suspicion of heatstroke.

Precautions to take when exercising in the heat

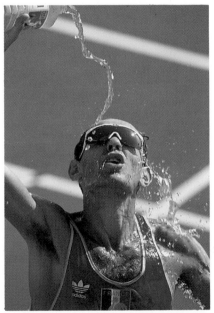

Clothing should be white, light weight, and loose fitting. Natural fibres are safer than synthetic ones. During endurance exercise small quantities of fluid should be drunk at frequent intervals and water sprayed on the skin at every opportunity. The use of sweat inhibiting deodorants should be avoided, and people should not exercise in the heat immediately after a glucose or high carbohydrate feed because blood is diverted from the skin into the gastrointestinal tract. Endurance events should be cancelled if the wet bulb/globe thermometer index exceeds 28°C.

After exercise

- Drinks should be cool but not iced.
- Showers should not be too cold because cold on the skin stimulates heat production and causes vasoconstriction thus reducing heat loss. People would stay hot and start sweating immediately after coming out of the shower and, at worst a cold shower might precipitate heatstroke. A safe and effective cooling method is to allow a cool shower to play over only the head, neck, hands, wrists, feet, and ankles.

Water on the skin can prevent overheating.

Effects of acclimatisation to heat

Increase in:	Decrease in:
Work output	Heart rate
Endurance	Pulse pressure
Plasma volume	Basal oxygen consumption
Sweat production	Sweat electrolyte concentration
	Skin and core temperature

Acclimatisation, which should be specific for the destination environment—that is, dry or humid heat—produces beneficial physiological changes.

Adaptation occurs over 10-14 days of heat exposure (the biggest changes in days 3-5), but is lost within a few weeks unless exposure to heat is repeated regularly at intervals of four days or less. Exercise training by itself is less effective than regular heavy exercise in the heat—for example, in a hot room or sauna or wearing an impermeable track suit.

The photographs are reproduced with permission of Allsport and Dr William J Mills Jnr, Anchorage, Alaska.

WATER SPORTS

J D M Douglas

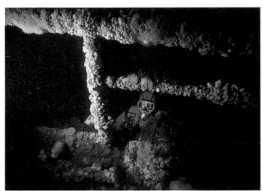

Diver at a wreck in UK waters.

Supervised training and instruction are the essence of safety for water sports. All outdoor adventure sports have predictable risks and survival techniques, which are best learned through clubs affiliated to their national organisations, such as the British Sub Aqua Club, Royal Yachting Association, British Canoe Union, Royal Yachting Association, and British Water Ski Federation. They produce statistics based on accident reports and modify training procedures if trends are noted. They all have honorary medical support.

Swimming

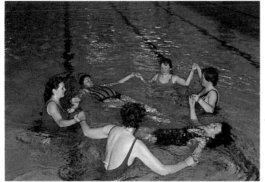

"Aqua-natal" class.

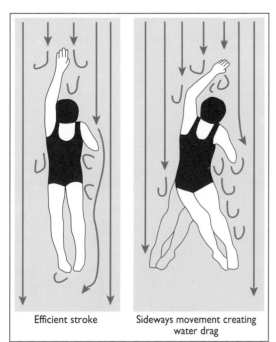

Efficient stroke | Sideways movement creating water drag

Swimming efficiency and front crawl: left—efficient stroke; right—sideways movement creating water drag.

Benefits and contraindications

Swimming is a physical activity that can be enjoyed safely by people at any age. Gentle swimming provides an injury free method of exercising joints and muscles. It is the ideal exercise to prevent and rehabilitate musculoskeletal injuries to the neck and back. Breast stroke requires repeat flexion and extension of the neck, whereas front crawl develops erector spinae, psoas, and latissmus dorsi. Patients with paraplegia gain confidence from the buoyancy given to weak limbs.

People who have had hip or knee replacements should avoid breast stroke because the frog leg kick risks dislocation. Those with multiple joint replacements should be advised that they may be negatively buoyant.

Antenatal water exercise

"Aqua-natal" classes are a new fashion in antenatal care, which should be encouraged and supported by doctors. Trained midwives supervise "water aerobics" to music while the pregnant women stand in a pool and use floating for relaxation. Participation can be encouraged (in swimmers and non-swimmers) from the first trimester to near term to help posture and breathing in a "weightless" environment. Postnatally babies can be reintroduced to swimming with care for their temperature from about 3 months. Children with grommets may swim on the surface from one month after insertion at the surgeon's discretion.

Oxygen uptake with different strokes

Comparative studies of oxygen uptake in triathletes suggest that speed is related to skill rather than aerobic power. The oxygen cost of swimming at a constant speed differs with strokes, front crawl being the most energy efficient.

Comparative oxygen uptake and heart rate in the same swimmer using different strokes at constant speed

Stroke	Speed (m/s)	Oxygen uptake (l/min)	Heart rate (beats/min)
Front crawl	1·0	1·83	125
Backstroke	1·0	2·42	138
Butterfly	1·0	2·85	150
Breaststroke	1·0	3·42	162

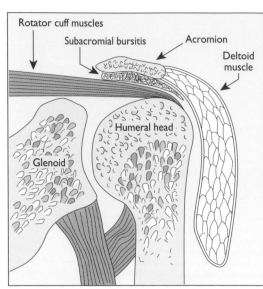

Crawl swimmers' shoulder. Repeated impingement of the humeral head into the overlying acromion.

Immersion and drowning

Cardiovascular fitness

Swimming improves cardiovascular fitness for healthy people but needs to be regular and vigorous; 20 minutes continuous swimming three times a week is ideal. A swimmer of average ability should be able to cover half a mile (32 lengths of a 25 metre pool) without stopping.

Cardiac rehabilitation—Heart rates during swimming are lower than during equivalent land based exercise, and venous return is encouraged by hydrostatic pressure. Patients can be encouraged to return to swimming six to eight weeks after myocardial infarction.

Special problems in competitive swimmers

Chlorine conjunctivitis can be prevented by wearing good goggles. *Chronic otitis externa* caused by bacterial or fungal infection in the macerated external ear canal can be treated topically with ear drops. Some swimmers find propylactic alcohol and acetic acid drops or ear plugs helpful. Bony exostosis of the external auditory meatus may require surgical removal.

Shoulder pain—Front crawl and butterfly stroke cause shoulder pain by repeated abduction followed by forced adduction. This movement requires the rotator cuff muscles to pull the humeral head under the acromium, which may result in subacromial bursitis or impingement syndrome. Treatment is rest with non-steroidal anti-inflammatory drugs or steroid injections into the subacromial bursa. The shoulder joint becomes unstable in back crawl and may partially dislocate with each stroke, which leads to tears of the cartilaginous rim of the glenoid socket. Avoiding using hand paddles and doing exercises to strengthen the rotator cuff muscles will help prevent this problem.

Knee pain in breast stroke results from the repeated valgus forces on the knee, which put a strain on the medial collateral ligament. Flexion and extension of the knee in all strokes can cause patella compression pain and chondromalacia patella. Quadriceps exercise and using neoprene knee braces during training may help.

Thermal protection

● Neoprene wet suits are worn in most water sports during the summer months throughout the UK and can increase survival times by up to 24 hours. An outer windproof shell garment increases their efficiency

● Dry suits are waterproof "bags" sealed at the neck and wrists. Thermal underclothing increases their efficiency for winter water sports, but they lose their buoyancy if punctured

● Survival advice for sailors in the water includes staying with the boat and, to conserve heat, adopting a fetal position and not swimming

● In boats, people should lie down to avoid wind chill and give priority to insulating the head and neck, as these are the areas of greatest heat loss once the circulation has adapted to cold stress

● Alcohol consumption is strongly associated with deaths from drowning and with cervical spine injuries resulting from diving into shallow water. It also potentiates cold stress by vasodilatation, hypoglycaemia, and mental confusion

---

Low water temperature

Outdoor water sports in the United Kingdom inland and coastal waters require planning to deal with voluntary or involuntary immersion in water from 0°C to 12°C. The thermal conductivity of water is 20 times that of air, and cooling occurs over time in water temperatures below 34°C. In cold water the body's outer shell attempts to protect the inner core temperature by peripheral vasoconstriction in the limbs, which makes them feel useless. Normal deep body temperature is 37°C; mental confusion, sleepiness, and loss of will to survive develop at 34°C core temperature. Unconsciousness at 30°C and ventricular fibrillation below 28°C lead to death at around 24°C.

Hypothermia—Channel swimmers survive because of their fat distribution. Adolescents seem to be particularly vulnerable to cold stress in water or on mountains because of their large surface area in proportion to their low body volume. Early symptoms of hypothermia include apathy and withdrawal. Sudden immersion in icecold water quickly incapacitates even very strong swimmers, with reflex tachycardia, hypertension, and hyperventilation sometimes leading to sudden death.

Hydrostatic pressure—Immersion exerts a hydrostatic squeeze on venous return. After prolonged immersion (only possible if a life jacket is worn) sudden release of the pressure by lifting the casualty in an upright position may lead to circulatory collapse. Rescue in the supine position is therefore recommended but may be impossible in practice.

Resuscitation—The dilemma for doctors in an outdoor environment is when to start chest compression. Severe hypothermia may produce an impalpable carotid pulse, and rough handling may precipitate ventricular fibrillation.

Swallowed or inhaled water

The stomach is usually full of water swallowed during near drowning. No attempt should be made to "empty the lungs" of water because the volumes aspirated are small. Restoring a heart beat, monitoring cardiac function, and administering high concentration oxygen are essential first aid measures. In hospital, the rectal temperature and an electrocardiogram should be taken before resuscitation is abandoned. Victims of near drowning who have inhaled water should be kept under observation for at least 24 hours in case pulmonary oedema develops.

Fresh or salt water

Management after immersion in fresh water is no different from that after salt water immersion.

Leptospirosis—Stagnant inland water may be contaminated by this spirochaete from rat or cattle urine. The presenting symptom is an illness like influenza that starts 7-12 days after exposure. The haemorrhagic complications of Weil's disease are prevented by early recognition and treatment with penicillin, erythromycin, or tetracycline. Cuts should be covered before immersion and showers taken afterwards. Doctors should be informed of the risk by the sports person.

Sport diving

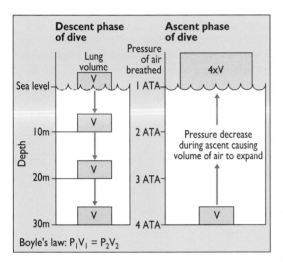

Boyle's law: $P_1V_1 = P_2V_2$

There are about 70 000 scuba divers in Britain. (Scuba stands for self contained underwater breathing apparatus.) Each year there are about 12 deaths and 70 episodes of decompression illness that require recompression. These should, however, be set against the several hundred thousand dives, which means that mortality and morbidity compares favourably with those for mountaineering, a sport with similar levels of risk and numbers of devotees.

Breathing compressed air during descent

To equalise the pressure in the body's air-filled cavities (sinuses, middle ear space, and lungs) divers breathe air from an aqualung at a pressure equal to that of the surrounding water. Water pressure increases by one atmosphere absolute (1 ATA or 1 bar) for every 10 metres of descent, and the gases behave according to the physical gas laws.

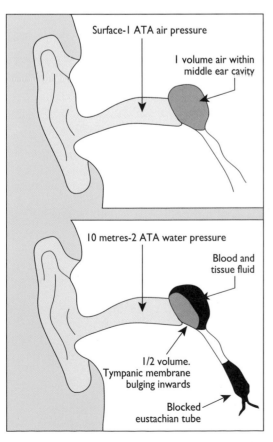

Blocking of a eustachian tube during descent will lead to aural barotrauma, which is the most common dysbaric illness. The bruising of the tympanic membrane should resolve within two weeks, and antibiotics are usually required. Perforations need to be healed completely before diving is resumed. Rarely, the inner ear also becomes damaged, causing an oval or round window perilymph leak. Tinnitus, vertigo, and deafness require urgent assessment by an ear, nose, and throat specialist.

Nitrogen narcosis

Nitrogen is highly soluble in fat and exerts a narcotic effect on the central nervous system as its partial pressure increases. At depths below 30 metres nitrogen narcosis has an effect similar to that of alcohol intoxication and is a serious hazard to personal safety. The resulting euphoria, overconfidence, poor mental judgement, and aggravation of panic are potentiated by drugs acting on the central nervous system, which are contraindicated in diving. Nitrogen narcosis resolves spontaneously without any hangover when the diver ascends to a shallower depth. Helium is much less soluble in fat and must be used to replace nitrogen at depth below 50 metres in commercial diving.

Acute decompression illness

Forms of onset	Manifestations
Progressive	Cutaneous
Static	Neurological
Relapsing	Cardiopulmonary
Spontaneous	Joint pain
	Constitutional

Acute decompression illness

Air in the lungs must be vented while divers surface because the expansion of gas volume predicted by Boyle's Law will result in pulmonary barotrauma if there is any attempt at breath holding or if a person has an air trapping disease. Cerebral arterial gas embolism, pneumothorax, or mediastinal emphysema can result from an uncontrolled ascent.

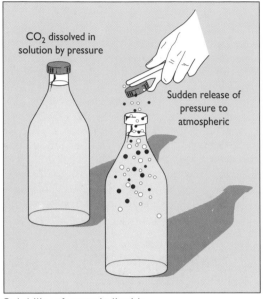

CO_2 dissolved in solution by pressure

Sudden release of pressure to atmospheric

Solubility of gases in liquids.

Nitrogen that has dissolved in body tissue during a dive must be excreted via the lungs during the ascent and after surfacing. Bubbles of nitrogen form in the tissues and blood if pressure is reduced too quickly. Gas trapped in soft tissues around a joint gives rise to shoulder or elbow pain and, when more widely disseminated in the body, to chest pains or neurological symptoms. Decompression illness can be reduced, but not eliminated, by using decompression stoppage tables or wrist-held diving computers to control ascents.

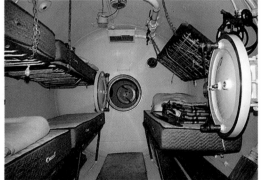

Inside of a recompression chamber.

Neurological symptoms occurring within 24 hours of surfacing must be considered to be a manifestation of acute decompression illness until proved otherwise. They must be treated urgently by recompression. Divers will usually describe chest pains within 10 minutes of surfacing; these resolve but proceed to a deep, boring, lumbar backache and girdle pains. Losses of feeling, motor power, and coordination of the legs can quickly proceed to permanent spinal paralysis. A diver who cannot walk or pass urine when in an accident and emergency department requires 100% oxygen and immediate transfer to a hyperbaric unit for recompression, after liaison with the unit about the means of transport. Air transport is quick, but altitude causes the bubbles to expand. Indeed, decompression illness may initially manifest itself after a flight home from a foreign diving holiday.

Emergency phone numbers for diving emergencies

HM Coastguard (via 999 or VHF Channel 16) provide communication links for all maritime emergencies

England and Wales:
Royal Navy: 01831 151523
Plymouth Area: 01752 261910

Scotland:
Aberdeen: 01224 681818

Ireland:
Craigavon: 01762 336711

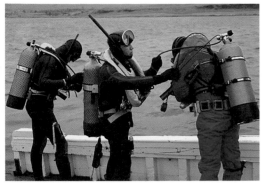

Safety relies on diving in pairs.

Diving safety

Medical examinations—The United Kingdom Sport Diving Medical Committee requires people to have a thorough medical examination before starting training with a club. The examination forms contain guidance for doctors and lists of voluntary medical referees to consult in doubtful cases.

Chronic illnesses—Improvement in the treatment and control of diabetes and asthma has allowed United Kingdom clubs to select and train people with these conditions. Diving accident statistics from Australia, however, suggest that a cautious approach is still required to prevent deaths in people with chronic illnesses. Epilepsy and drugs acting on the central nervous system remain contraindications to sport diving.

Training—Good basic training within a recognised club remains the cornerstone of diving safety.

Other water sports

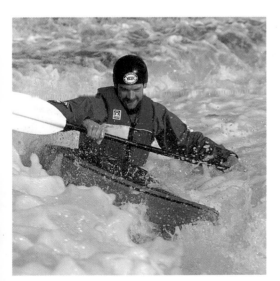

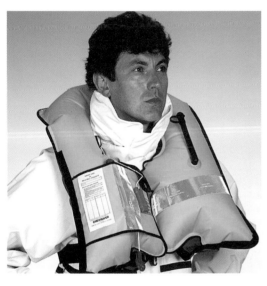

Canoeing

Helmets are required in white water canoeing because head injury is an obvious risk. Anterior dislocation of the shoulder can be caused by extreme high brace manoeuvres. Wrist tenosynovitis can occur in long distance kayaking but is prevented by cranked paddle handles and angled blades.

Sailing and board sailing

Competitive dinghy and board sailing required prolonged tension in the abdominal, quadriceps, and back leg muscles to balance the wind forces. Anterior knee pain can also occur in young dinghy sailors with chondromalacia patellas.

Standing in the wind, repeated immersion, and exertion make board sailors at risk of exhaustion and hypothermia.

In yachts an unexpected movement of the main sail (involuntary gybe) may cause serious head injury or sweep a sailor overboard. Clothing, safety lines, and life jackets should be planned in advance of changing weather conditions. Cold stress is serious in combination with prolonged seasickness; cinnarazine tablets or hyoscine patches are popular prophylacytic measures against seasickness.

Water skiing

Propeller and impact injuries are an obvious risk but can be prevented by following boat safety procedures and by wearing helmets for ski jumping. Serious injury has been caused by water douching into the vagina or rectum during ski jumping, but this can be prevented by wearing a wet suit.

Rowing

Rowing is a safe sport with a low injury rate, but it can cause low back pain and tenosynovitis of the wrist.

A new European standard specifies the correct choice of life jacket or buoyancy aid for different applications. Top: a life jacket must self-right an unconscious non-swimmer but may be uncomfortable to wear or require the maintenance of CO_2 cylinders. Bottom: buoyancy aids are a safe alternative, giving freedom of movement during sport and once immersed. Wet suits are also buoyant.

The author gratefully acknowledges advice from the Royal Yachting Association, British Canoe Union, British Water Ski Federation, British Olympic Medical Centre, and Mr C Howie.

The table showing oxygen uptake with different swimming strokes and the drawings showing efficiency of front crawl and crawl swimmers' shoulder are reproduced with permission from Blackwell Scientific Publications.

SPORT AND EXERCISE PSYCHOLOGY

Nanette Mutrie

Sport and exercise psychology is concerned with observing, explaining, predicting, and perhaps changing behaviours in competitive and recreational environments. It is an applied psychology (like industrial psychology and educational psychology) and does not rely on any one theoretical position (such as behavioural or cognitive psychology) to derive applications. At the competitive end of this range of application (sport psychology) are issues such as preparing elite athletes psychologically to perform at their best or understanding why so many talented youngsters drop out of sport. At the recreational end (exercise psychology) are issues such as how to increase the percentage of the population who are physically active and finding ways to help patients adhere to their "exercise prescription."

Sport psychology

Simple physical development alone is no guarantee of success in sport; a performer must also have the right mental "set"—that is, the fine tuning of the brain—for performance. This could make all the difference between an adequate performance and an excellent one.

National Coaching Foundation

National Coaching Foundation courses in sport psychology

Introductory level:	Mind over matter
Key course level:	Motivating your athlete
	Mental preparation for performance
	Understanding and improving skill
Advanced workshop:	Mental training

The role of psychology in sports performance is clearly recognised by coaches, athletes, spectators, and journalists. Interviews after events often show that success or failure has been attributed to psychological aspects of performance; "the team were not motivated today," "I could not feel the rhythm," "I was very focused, nothing could distract me," are common quotations. As technical and physical preparation advances, there is little to separate winners from losers. The role of psychology in performance has therefore become more important. People used to believe that the psychological attributes that are important for success in sport were innate; athletes either had these skills, or they did not. However, the theoretical and research base in sport psychology has developed considerably in parallel with the growth of sport science in general. Many elite squads of athletes currently have a sport psychologist working with them to assist in learning appropriate psychological skills. The National Coaching Foundation (NCF) includes psychological topics in coach education programmes in recognition that the coach must know about psychological aspects of performance in order to guide athletes appropriately. It is important to educate coaches about these psychological issues because not everyone has access to, or will want to work with, a sport psychologist. Ideally, athletes should learn psychological skills alongside the technical skills of their sport.

Maximising performance has clearly attracted the most attention in sport psychology but extensive publications exist on other topics, such as maintaining motivation and avoiding drop out from sport requiring motor skills, the psychophysiology of successful performance, and the social psychology of sport.

The theoretical models of sport psychology have often been adapted from mainstream psychology. For example, it has recently been suggested that the "inverted U" hypothesis, which suggests that optimal performance will occur with moderate levels of arousal, needs refinement before it can be applied to sports performance. In this model arousal refers to physiological indices such as breathing rate, heart rate, sweating response, muscle tension, and brain wave patterns. Some sports (such as sprinting) require very high levels of arousal for best performance whereas others (such as archery) require very low levels of arousal for best performance. In addition, arousal levels are possibly only part of the issue and anxiety levels (that is, the extent to which an athlete has doubts, fears, or worries) should probably also be taken into account. Researchers continue to adapt, refine, or create

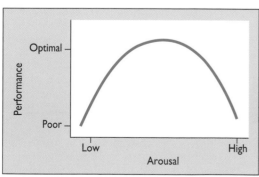

Inverted U hypothesis of the relation between arousal and performance in sport. Does this fully explain performance in sport?

theoretical models for sport psychology, while practitioners select and apply the techniques that can help athletes deal with some of the common sports problems. One important point for all of these techniques is that they must be rehearsed. Ideally coaches should provide time in most training sessions to address psychological skills and athletes may also have to practise certain skills (such as progressive muscular relaxation) off the field of play.

Anxiety control

Many performers do well in practice but find it difficult to perform at their best in competition. Some aspect of the competition—the crowd, the expectations, the importance of the event—increases the athlete's anxiety levels. This can result in excess muscle tension (somatic anxiety), lack of confidence (cognitive anxiety), and failure to perform at his or her best. Techniques that can be used to help control anxiety levels include:

● The use of questionnaires designed to help the athlete and coach assess the kind of anxiety that is present. Records of performance have to be noted alongside the assessments as anxiety is mainly a problem when it has been shown to upset performance; some athletes may be at their best when they feel "nervous"

● Teaching relaxation skills, such as progressive muscular relaxation or transcendental meditation, to control the symptoms of anxiety

● Teaching cognitive skills, such as positive self-statements, visualisation, and thought-stopping, to help athletes control their cognitive anxiety.

Confidence building

Techniques that can enhance confidence include setting goals, learning a positive approach to competition, and creating a practice environment that does not constantly undermine self esteem. Goal setting teaches athletes to plan ahead, to analyse the main improvements required for success, and to set goals that are both realistic and challenging; it has been shown to be an effective motivational tool. When athletes note successes in their short term goals the intermediate and long term goals seem more in their reach.

Concentration training

Being unable to focus on the task in hand, because the crowd, the referee, the opposition, or one's own thought processes have created a distraction, is a common problem for athletes. Concentration skills can be improved by identifying the common distractions for an athlete and mentally rehearsing a plan of how to bring attention back to where it is required. For example, a tennis player who is distracted by apparently poor line calls can rehearse letting that frustration go and focus on producing good form in the next shot to be played.

Dealing with teams

Dealing with the varying personalities and motivations of a team of players and creating a cohesive unit is one of the most difficult tasks of a coach, team manager, or team captain. A suggested model of team cohesion differentiates between the perception of bonding within the group (group integration) and the attraction of individuals to the group. In addition, the model shows that cohesion is related both to the social interactions of the group and to the tasks of the group (that is, what the team would like to achieve in terms of performance). A questionnaire has been developed to assess these aspects of cohesion. Various possible techniques for enhancing team cohesion include creating an environment in which everyone has a chance to voice an opinion, avoiding the formation of cliques, and teaching athletes to appreciate each other's qualities.

Other aspects of working with teams include understanding how groups develop, selecting the correct "leader," and communication within the group. Knowledge of the principles of group dynamics is important.

Re-focus plan example

Distractions(s)
Official gives poor line calls

Cues
Take a deep breath, exhale slowly
Walk to position
Focus on grip and stance for next shot

GOAL SETTING CHART
(for week beginning . . .)

LONG TERM GOAL

INTERMEDIATE GOALS		Date
1	by	
2	by	
3	by	

SHORT TERM GOALS THIS WEEK

☐ 1

☐ 2

☐ 3

☐ 4

☐ 5

☐ 6

☐ 7

Tick if achieved

Conceptual model of group cohesion (Widmeyer, Brawley, and Carron, 1985).

Sport and exercise psychology

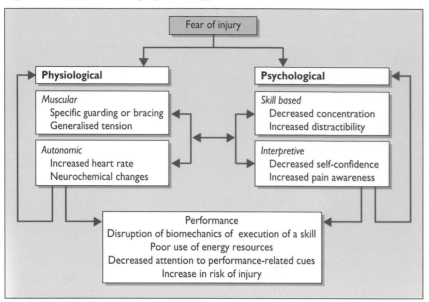

The mind and body connection: a psychophysiological model of risk (Heil, 1993).

Injured athletes

The basic techniques of sport psychology possibly can be used to enhance recovery from an injury. When athletes experience an injury they may become depressed, believing that they will lose training time or that they may never perform at their previous level again. A holistic approach to injury rehabilitation, which includes the mental rehearsal of the skills that cannot be physically practised and the physical training of uninjured parts of the body, should be adopted. In addition, relaxation skills may help in the recovery process by reducing unwanted muscle tension, and positive imagery of returning to the scenario in which the injury occurred may help build confidence. Physiological and psychological factors may interact to create fear of injury in athletes. Awareness of these factors could help to predict those most at risk of being injured.

Exercise psychology

Spend a few minutes writing out two lists; one containing the possible GAINS from your participation in exercise and the other containing the possible LOSSES from participation in exercise

GAINS	LOSSES
——————————	——————————
——————————	——————————
——————————	——————————
——————————	——————————

If you have listed more gains than losses this should reinforce your commitment to the exercise programme. Whenever you feel like missing out an exercise session you should think about these positive benefits.

If you have listed more losses than gains then it is unlikely that you will stick to your exercise programme. Look again at the losses. Can you overcome them? Can you find more gains?

Exercise psychology is a newer discipline than sport psychology. It has evolved from the need for a psychological perspective on the message that exercise is good for health. From this perspective two particular sub-themes have emerged—namely, exercise adherence and psychological outcomes of activity.

Exercise adherence

Exercise adherence refers to a range of topics concerned with getting the general population to be more physically active. The Allied Dunbar National Fitness Survey showed that 7/10 men and 8/10 women were below the threshold level of activity that could provide health benefits, and up to 50% of people who begin an exercise programme for health are thought to drop out within the first six months. The questions are how to motivate people to start more physical activity, how to overcome perceived barriers to activity, and how to maintain activity on a regular basis throughout life. Exercise adherence is also important for patients who have been advised to exercise to improve a medical condition (such as diabetes, asthma, obesity, osteoporosis, and in cardiac rehabilitation.) Techniques to help adherence include setting appropriate exercise goals, time management, and building support from friends and family.

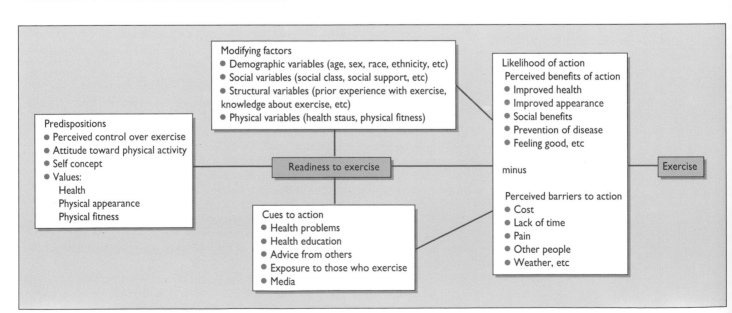

The exercise behaviour model (Widmeyer, Brawley and Carron, 1985).

Sports council research strategy in sport psychology

Motivation
  Dynamics of motivation
  Reasons for the pursuit of dangerous sports
  Role of attributions in sport
  Coach and performer burnout

Motor control and learning
  Role of cognition in motor control
  Direct links of perception and action in the skilful control of actions
  Hierarchical models of motor control

Stress and performance
  Pre-competitive emotional states
  Relation of stress to performance

Group dynamics
  Leadership and decision making styles
  Influence of group cohesion, social support, and other related variables on performance

Excellence and wellbeing
  Psychosocial factors in proneness to injury and psycho-immunosuppression
  Psychology of the injured athlete
  Moral development and the pursuit of excellence

Psychological skills training and consultancy work
  Mechanisms and processes underlying the effects of psychological skills training
  Factors that influence adherence to psychological skills training
  Evaluation of clients' needs and sport psychologists' effectiveness
  Examination of the various roles that might need to be assumed by effective practising sport psychologists

Psychological outcomes

How physical activity relates to mental wellbeing has not been extensively researched. Current knowledge suggests that advantages of physical activity include improved mood, increased ability to cope with stress, and enhanced self esteem. Work has shown that exercise can alleviate moderate levels of depression and anxiety and can enhance the effects of treatment in cardiac and alcohol rehabilitation. The reason is not yet clear but the mechanism is probably more complex than a "fitness effect" as some psychological benefits have been noted without apparent improvement in fitness. The popular press has supported the idea that neurotransmitters such as endorphins are responsible for feeling better after exercise or even for becoming dependent on exercise. The plasma endorphin levels after exercise have, however, proved difficult to link with the mood enhancing effects of exercise. Further research is required to establish how the physiological and psychological changes that occur as a result of exercise explain the positive changes noted in these patients.

Who provides sport and exercise psychology?

The conceptual model of group cohesion is reprinted from Carron, *Group Dynamics in Sport*, 1988, Spodym Publishers. The exercise behaviour model are reprinted with permission of *Health Education* and the psychophysiological model of risk with permission of *Psychology of Sport Injury*.

In the United Kingdom the British Association of Sport and Exercise Sciences (BASES) has an accreditation procedure for sport psychologists. Accreditation is given to those who have the necessary educational qualifications and have had sufficient supervised practice. Many coaches have taken courses on the subject, team doctors with a diploma in sports medicine will have studied psychology, and most people with a sport or exercise science degree will have some knowledge of psychological issues. The National Coaching Foundation (NCF) provides courses at four levels, and both the NCF and the Scottish Sports Council have distance learning material about sports psychology.

PHYSIOTHERAPY FOR SPORTS INJURIES

Vivian Grisogono

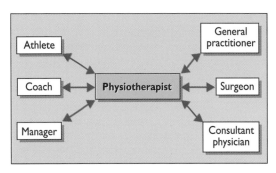

Sports physiotherapists have to be sensitive and sympathetic to injured players' longing to be back in action immediately. Equally, patients have to be restrained from taking short cuts that could lead to further short term or long term harm.

In all circumstances the aims of physiotherapy treatment are to relieve pain, reduce swelling, promote healing, improve strength and mobility, and restore full physical function. Treatments include manipulation, massage, electrotherapy, hydrotherapy, and exercise therapy.

Physiotherapists are often the first contacts of injured athletes and so may see patients without referral from a medical practitioner. Sports physiotherapists always, however, act as part of a team. Contact is normally maintained with a patient's general practitioner, and with other medical and paramedical staff as necessary. Ideally, general practitioners faced with any sports injury that does not require medical or surgical care will *always* refer the patient for physiotherapy treatment or guidance from a physiotherapist, or both. Part of the physiotherapist's role is to act as a link between the athlete, coach, and manager on one side and the medical team on the other.

Manual therapy for sports injuries

Massage

Chartered (qualified) physiotherapists are trained in all the techniques relevant to sports injuries. Massage is an essential element in sports physiotherapy. It can be used prophylactically, to help reduce muscle tightness and tension after hard sessions, or to improve muscle tone and the circulation as part of the warm up before a training session or a competition. For injuries massage is used, gently in the first instance, to help promote healing by improving the local blood flow, to relieve muscular spasm, and to reduce swelling.

One of the advantages of using massage is that experienced physiotherapists can feel the state of the injured tissues, and also the tissue response to the treatment. Different massage techniques are used for different purposes: for instance, slow movements using medium pressure relax the tissues, whereas deep frictions create a harsher effect and might be used for stimulation, especially in chronic tendon conditions.

There are, of course, circumstances in which massage should be used with caution, if at all. This applies specially to muscle haematomas, particularly in large muscle groups such as the quadriceps, where deep massage directly over a haematoma may promote myositis ossificans.

Manipulation

Manipulation is identified with passive joint movement, and can be closely associated with massage. The mildest form of manipulation consists of gentle oscillating movements over a joint, usually described as Maitland's techniques. At the other end of the scale are full thrust, or grade 5, manipulations in which one or more joints are forced through their most extreme range of movement.

Any of the body's moving joints can be manipulated or mobilised by passive movement. The aim of manipulation is to relieve pain, improve localised circulation, and increase joint range. For injured sports people (and any other patient), however, manipulation or mobilisation techniques have to be matched with remedial exercises. Increasing joint range without strengthening the protective muscle groups leaves the joint potentially unstable.

Aims of massage
- To reduce muscle tightness and tension
- To improve muscle tone and circulation
- To promote healing of injuries
- To relieve muscle spasm
- To reduce swelling

Aims of manipulation
- To relieve pain
- To improve localised circulation
- To increase joint range

Active rehabilitation

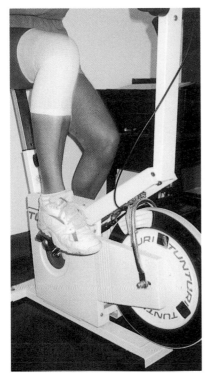

Exercise treatment: using a static bicycle with saddle lowered to improve knee flexion.

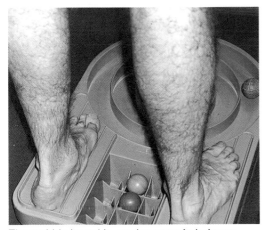

The wobble board is used to re-train balance mechanisms after any leg injury, especially ankle sprains.

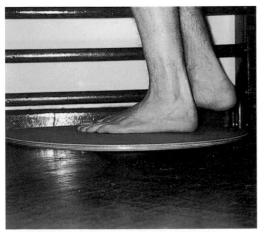

Dynamic strengthening and proprioceptive exercise for the legs using the wobbler.

Exercise treatment

Of all the treatment methods, exercise therapy is the most vital. Injured sports players need to be shown accurate remedial exercises in relation to any injury. Alongside these, an alternative fitness training schedule has to be set out, with due regard for the capacities of the patient, the restrictions of the injury, and the requirements for his or her sport.

Inhibition

Inhibition is the direct result of any injury in any part of the body. If damaged tissue heals without the associated recovery of active movement in or around the injured area then the inhibition remains, so the patient will use compensatory movement. In many cases the compensation needed may only be very slight, but it always interferes with normal patterns of movement, which creates selective weakness or tightness. This may ultimately contribute to repeat injury or to secondary injury in a related area.

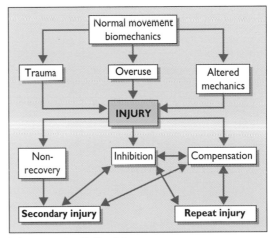

Injury: a potentially vicious sequence.

Isometric exercises

In the first stages of injury isometric exercises, or movements within a very small range, may be the only type of strengthening work the patient can achieve without pain. These exercises are essential after injuries to joints, especially to the knee, spine, or shoulder. If possible the isometric exercises are combined with active movements for joints that relate to the injured part—for instance, hip abduction and extension movements with the knee locked into extension are used as quickly as possible after any knee injury.

Coordination

Coordination is the ultimate goal of any remedial exercise programme for rehabilitation after a sports injury. It is not just a question of gaining pain relief and localised activity in the injured area but also of restoring proper interaction between the injured part and the areas around it. For this reason one of the most valuable exercise tools for any leg injury is the wobble board, which can be used to re-train all the proprioceptive nerve systems.

Physiotherapy for sports injuries

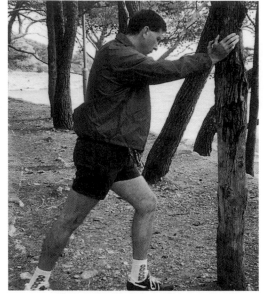

Passive stretching exercises are vital for improving flexibility after injury, and they should be used subsequently in the athlete's warm up and warm down routines.

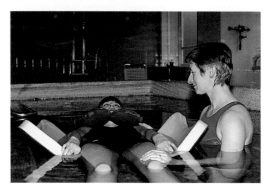

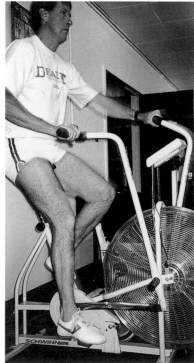

The Airdyne static bicycle provides coordinated activity for the arms and legs.

Passive stretching

Passive stretching exercises are usually used from an early stage to restore flexibility within an injured muscle or round an injured joint. The stretched position is held absolutely still, within painless limits, then relaxed, before the stretch is repeated. To increase joint range, bouncing type mobilising movements may be used. In most cases strengthening exercises are used alongside the stretching or mobilising work, to avoid instability.

Hydrotherapy

Exercise in a hydrotherapy pool can be a useful part of a rehabilitation programme. It can be used at an early stage to mobilise patients after severe trauma or after surgery such as laminectomy. Specialist hydrotherapy pools are very warm to promote relaxation and the circulation and so encourage freedom of movement. A normal swimming pool can also be used for generalised exercises and alternative aerobic training.

Specific exercises

In the later stages of recovery, strengthening exercises within the painless range of muscle or joint movement are used, with special emphasis on eccentric muscle work. The exercises have to be executed precisely—for instance, in shoulder injury patients usually have to practise arm abduction movements while concentrating on eliminating any undue tension or contraction in the trapezius muscle.

Coordination exercises

In the final phase of recovery patients progress to coordinated actions, usually incorporating movements related to their sports, such as shadow strokes for racket games players or sprinting and turning for footballers or hockey players. The rehabilitation process should lead naturally to a patient's return to sport. In professional sports fitness tests are used mainly to boost the confidence of the player, coach, and manager. If the recovery programme has been properly completed, however, there should be no doubt that the player is fit again.

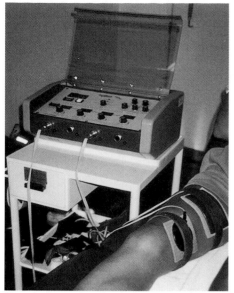

Electrical muscle stimulation to re-educate vastus medialis muscle.

Electrical muscle stimulation

To help precision in remedial exercises, the most useful electrotherapy is electrical muscle stimulation. Faradism is still useful as a self help treatment at home (after instruction) or in the absence of an updated machine. Modern electrical muscle stimulators still use a simple low frequency alternating current: their sophistication lies in providing variable frequencies, surges, pulse durations, and rest phases.

Re-educating normal muscle activity by electrical stimulation is especially useful when inhibition is a specific cause of a problem—such as in patellofemoral joint problems.

Electrical muscle stimulation may also be used at a very early stage after surgery or injury, even before active exercises are possible.

Slow pulse electrical muscle stimulation is a specific treatment for conditions such as compartment syndrome, in which there is hypertrophy or swelling in a fast muscle.

Pain relief, healing, and protection

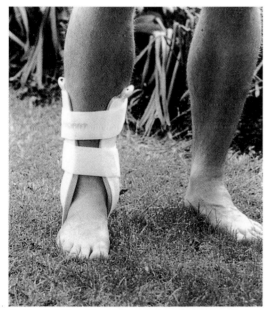

Ankle stabilised by stirrup splint (Aircast), which protects the joint while permitting a degree of functional movement.

Relieving pain and swelling

The pain of a sports injury can usually be well controlled with appropriate drugs. Physiotherapy techniques for relieving pain and any associated swelling include massage, ice applications (cryotherapy), ultrasonography, laser, diadynamic currents, interferential therapy, and pulsed short wave. Physiotherapists have to know when not to apply a given technique. For instance, ultrasound is best used in the very earliest stages of any injury, and its beneficial effects are known only in relation to a few specific types of tissue damage. Ultrasound may not be appropriate for chronic injuries, muscle tears, or possible stress problems in bone.

Early movement

It is well accepted that early movement, when possible, promotes healing after an injury. Even when a ruptured tissue has to be immobilised to permit good union, activating the uninjured tissues around it is still possible and necessary. After Achilles tendon rupture, for instance, sound functional union and high intensity alternative training is made possible by using taping and a removable cast. This treatment regimen avoids the problems of muscle wasting that is caused by immobilisation in a plaster cast and is thus a viable alternative to the previously passive version of conservative treatment. It can also be used postoperatively, providing especially good results after the Achilles has been sutured using the Ma technique.

Immobilisation

Taping (strapping) is used to protect injured areas while they need immobilisation. Any taping that encloses a joint and restricts movement also interferes with the coordination of an area. It is therefore especially important not to let a patient take part in stressful activities that would not be possible without the support. When support is needed to protect a joint from excess stress when it is just recovering from an injury, and perhaps also to boost a patient's confidence, the taping is usually applied locally rather than round the whole joint. The aim is to enhance the joint's proprioceptive system. For instance stirrup splints rather than complete taping may be used for the ankle.

Prophylactic taping to protect joints is much more widely used in the United States than in Britain, where the emphasis is much more on protective exercises and good background conditioning training than on restrictive supports.

Conclusion

Role of the sports physiotherapist

1) Creating a good patient relationship by being:
- Sensitive, sympathetic, caring, encouraging, yet persuasive, and firm

2) Preventing injury by:
- Giving advice on training, body conditioning, and protective exercises
- Prophylactic treatment

3) Treating injury using appropriate methods including:Ò
- Manipulation
- Massage
- Electrotherapy
- Hydrotherapy
- Exercise therapy

4) Ensuring safe return to training and competition by:
- Monitoring progress to full fitness
- Preventing a return to full activities too soon

The role of sports physiotherapists is to provide the necessary framework in which injured athletes can recover full fitness. Athletes need encouragement, sympathy, careful handling, and positive guidance. Successful rehabilitation and preventing repeat injury depend on an accurate and complete remedial exercise programme combined with suitable alternative fitness training.

The physiotherapist's role encompasses preventing as well as treating injury. Physiotherapists are not only vital members of medical back up teams for sports participants, but are also able to advise on protective exercises and safe training for sports players of every kind and level, from Olympic stars to joggers and keep-fitters.

THE COACH'S ROLE

Sue Campbell

Sport participants tend to fall into two categories—those who play for fun and recreation and those who are in the "serious" business of sports performance.

The first group often play sport to get fit, rather than get fit to play sport. They are likely to suffer a range of strains and pains which they may bring to their general practitioner, and need simple guidance on fitness principles. Positive preventive advice should reduce the incidence of injury.

Coaches have a vital role in the medical management of both groups. Courses in sports medicine for coaches have been organised at a number of levels by the National Coaching Foundation and are available throughout the United Kingdom. The introductory course is aimed at novice coaches and addresses basic principles, including the responsibilities of the coach in preventing injury, immediate treatment of injury, and the continuing care of the fit or injured athlete. The second level is aimed at club level coaches and was developed by the National Coaching Foundation, the Scottish Sports Council, and the St Andrew's Ambulance Association, and covers the complete range of injury from simple bruising to potentially life threatening situations.

Finally, an advanced course for senior experienced coaches helps to define the relationship of the coach to medical staff when dealing with performers who are ill or injured. It helps the coach to identify the signs and symptoms of injury or illness. The role of the coach in fitness testing and rehabilitation is also considered in some detail.

Help at the scene

Early effective treatment of injuries can ensure a much faster recovery. Recreational players have little in the way of immediate medical assistance available. At the very least, all sports clubs should have a full first aid kit available and access to emergency services. Often the first person at the scene of the incident is the coach and she or he needs to know what to do. Many recreational players simply rest until the injury heals; some may visit their local general practitioner. The more serious competitor will want treatment as quickly as possible as every day away from training can be vital when preparing for major competition.

Sports injuries clinics have been established in many towns. Doctors working in them usually have a special interest in sports medicine. The newly formed National Sports Medicine Institute is monitoring the quality of these services. Many local authorities are keen to establish sports injuries clinics and doctors hold a central role.

Doctor and coach relationship

It is often during treatment that the coach and doctor meet. Establishing a good working relationship is vital. Mutual respect and understanding between coach and

---

> **Objectives for the doctor and coach relationship**
> ● To develop a mutual trust and understanding between doctors, coaches, and athletes, so that each group has appropriate expectations
> ● To integrate theory and practice so that relevant problems are addressed
> ● To ensure quality of service through control of practice

doctor is important if the athlete is to receive proper guidance. A general fitness programme should be maintained during recovery from injury. It is better to take a little longer to return to full activity than to risk a recurrence. The coach may wish to put the athlete into competition before he or she is ready because of the pressure to produce a result, and this can sometimes be an area of conflict between doctor, coach, and athlete. Fitness assessment before returning to full training and competition is a part of rehabilitation.

Athletes often lose confidence when they are injured. This is a particular problem for those who get injured a second time, especially if this is due to poorly supervised treatment and training.

Athletes, whatever their sport and irrespective of whether or not they are paid, are becoming increasingly professional in their attitude to training and competition. There are few, if any, events where the traditional ethos of the amateur approach of turning up to compete is compatible with success at high level. This has led to an increased demand for help and advice over and above that traditionally provided by the coach. The advent of the support team (physiologist, nutritionist, psychologist, biomechanist, doctor, and physiotherapist), working with the coach towards the goal of improved performance, has become an accepted and necessary part of sport.

Conclusion

Recreational athletes, serious performers, and coaches require medical support. The priority is the development of a relationship between doctors, coaches, and athletes based on mutual trust, understanding, and respect for one another's skills. The medical contribution to health, active lifestyles, and the achievement of excellence cannot be underestimated. What is needed is a network of sports medicine centres at local level providing information, education, and treatment. These could then be linked with the National Coaching Foundation's 16 regional centres and the British Association of Sport and Exercise Sciences' accredited laboratories and individuals. This combination of coaching, sports science, and sports medicine must then begin to provide the kind of support needed to ensure that everyone taking part in sport, whatever their level, achieves maximum satisfaction and enjoyment.

The coach's role

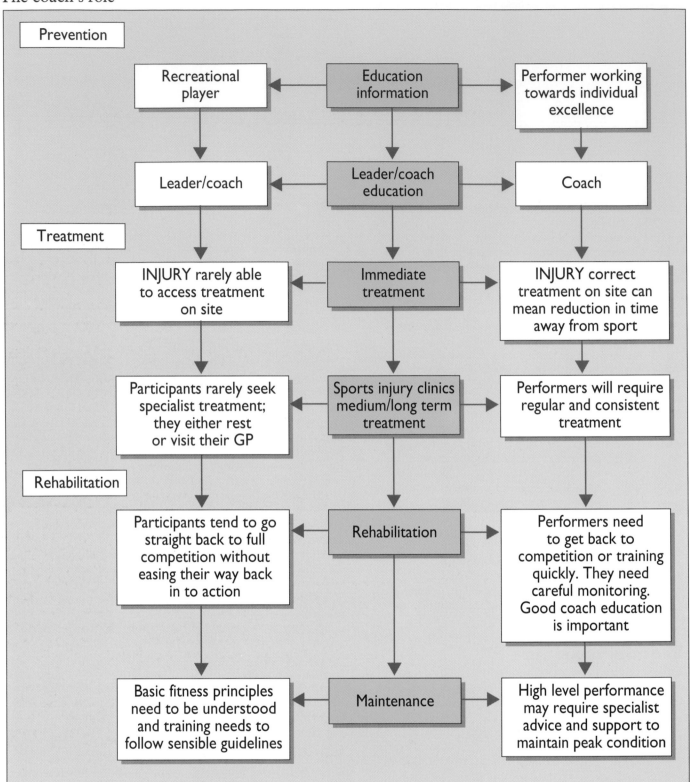

Roles of sports medicine experts

MEDICAL COVER FOR MAJOR SPORTING EVENTS

D S Tunstall-Pedoe

Medical hazards of major sporting events

Participants

- Trauma
- Hyperthermia
- Dehydration
- Exhaustion
- Hypothermia
- Hypoglycaemia

Spectators

- Secondary hazards—for example, motorcar or motorcycle racing and rallying, flying displays
- Hazards from being part of a large crowd, from each other, the stadium, and possibly even from police action—for example, riot, panic and crowd stampede, injuries from missiles, stabbing, trampling, suffocation, and fire
- Routine medical problems—for example, fits, faints, strokes, heart attacks, etc
- Medical problems caused by an unaccustomed environment—for example, sunburn, heat exhaustion, lightning strike, anaphylaxis from bee or wasp sting, etc

---

Medical organisation of large sports events is designed to prevent sudden overload of local ambulance and hospital facilities by spectators or competitors with minor problems that can be dealt with by first aiders. There should also be facilities for treating problems specific to the event.

Events can be regarded as major spectator events or major participant events, depending on whether the spectators (for example, in golf tournaments, football matches) or the participants (for example, in major road races) are likely to contribute the most casualties.

Major spectator events

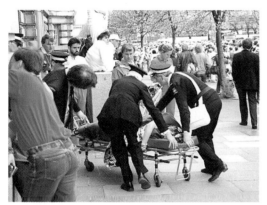

St John Ambulance Brigade stretcherbearers wheel a collapsed London marathon runner to the finish medical area.

Large crowds are the main concern. The venue should be covered by first aiders with ambulances and a medical room, or tent. Medical staff can deal with problems such as faints, fits, myocardial infarction, minor trauma, wasp sting, etc. Good communications and transport is essential where medical and first aid staff and facilities may be thinly spread.

Cardiac resuscitation should be available for any crowd larger than 30 000. First aid organisations such as St John Ambulance Brigade and the Red Cross have considerable experience of large crowds and are a ready source of advice.

Ideally one medical team should look after the crowd and another the athletes so that loyalties are not divided. Sports clubs often have their own physiotherapist and medical officer.

Protection of the crowd

Regulations on crowd control vary from sport to sport and from country to country. These have been tightened up as a result of various disasters in recent years, particularly the Hillsborough football stadium disaster.

Major participation events

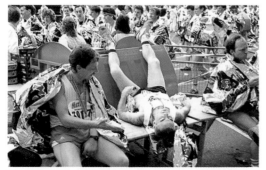

Runners recovering from the London marathon. A raised pelvis counteracts post race hypotension. Runners can easily become cold as space blankets give a false sense of security.

Major marathons, fun runs, triathlons, skiathlons, skating events and the like, which attract several thousand participants, pose a much greater challenge. The most famous are the marathons such as the London and New York marathons with as many as 25 000 runners on the day. The Great North Run in Newcastle, a half marathon, has even more participants, as do road races held over shorter distances in the United States. Numbers have exceeded 50 000 in these races and often the official field of registered runners is more than matched by a large number of "rogue" or "pirate" runners who have not registered and just turn up on the day, potentially swamping the organisation.

Major winter sports events can attract equally large numbers of participants and cover courses of 30, 50, or even 100 km of difficult terrain. In Britain charity cycle rides, such as the British Heart Foundation London to Brighton cycle ride (93 km), attract large numbers of cyclists of variable proficiency

These events all have their own logistical and medical problems and it is essential that there is a medical director, appointed early in the planning cycle. Reliance purely on late recruitment of a first aid organisation with little awareness of the likely problems is potentially dangerous. Medical care cannot be tacked on at the last minute to a major event.

Role of the medical director

Essential components for medical organisation

- A system of casualty collection and triage to deal with possible large numbers of casualties, often with trivial problems, most of which can be dealt with by proficient first aiders
- Ensuring that appropriate and sufficient medical expertise is available where needed, probably by a system of first aid posts and a field hospital or medical tent with cots and chairs, so that casualties can be dealt with rapidly
- Adequate communications, not only for the efficient collection, management and evacuation of casualties, but also so that there is accurate information available to relatives and friends
- Ambulance availability and access so that casualties can be evacuated from any part of the course without major disruption of the event

Other aspects of organisation

Competitors' numbers—useful for identification but not infallible, as they may give their registered number to a friend

Medical records—Statistics on the event are only as accurate as the data recorded but are essential for future planning. Individual medical records should be subject to medical confidentiality. Medical cards may have to be designed specifically for the event

The media—There needs to be agreement on what access is given to the press and television. They should not normally have access to medical areas, but should have ready access to the medical director to discuss medical problems

Local hospitals—These should be warned of the event, given advice on how to deal with special problems, and given advice on how to contact the medical director to discuss problems (such as how to reunite hospital casualties with their clothes, money, and relatives). Hospitals should also be asked to make their own medical records on competitors accessible to the medical director

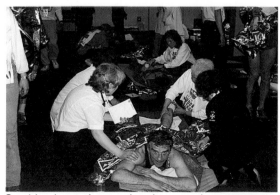

Combined attention to a London marathon runner at the finish from St John Ambulance Brigade staff and a physiotherapist.

The medical director should have a close involvement with the sport. His or her opinion is more likely to be respected if he or she is a former competitor. The medical director is a "figurehead," essential for press liaison and speedy answers to questions posed by the event organisers, a role not easily filled by a medical committee with no defined leader. The medical director should attend planning meetings for the event and be kept fully involved in discussions wherever safety and the welfare of the participants is involved. He or she may be required or wish to give advice on entry to the event (for example, suitable ages, whether any medical certification of fitness is required to compete) and frequency and location of aid and refreshment points.

The course and projected timing of the event (if it is likely to be very hot) must be safe for the participants. They should receive in advance of the event appropriate medical advice about training and participation, by direct mailing (see below) and through newspaper articles in the local press (and television). He or she should ensure that there is nutritional support: water and sports drinks along the course, and food and drink available at the finish. Rapid access for participants to their clothes and other belongings is also important.

Staffing and medical support

Volunteers can be used to man aid stations, with groups of doctors and nurses supported by radio hams and (in the United States) state troopers with army ambulances. In Britain it is usual to make use of the expertise of the voluntary first aid organisations—St John Ambulance Brigade, the Red Cross, or St Andrew's Ambulance Association.

These organisations can supply highly disciplined groups of first aiders and some doctors and nurses, but above all they have experience of large events and have ambulances and communications and close liaison with the police. Individual staff may not have had experience of particular events, so briefing lectures and first aid advice sheets from the medical director as well as close liaison with the first aid organisation of choice is required.

Aid posts and ambulances

Problems arise when vehicles such as ambulances and groups of personnel are placed or moved around without agreement of all the parties concerned. It is essential that the event medical director, event director, and first aid organisation senior officer work amicably together and with the police and agree on the siting of aid points and ambulances. Any changes made to agreed plans must be justified and agreed by all parties. The police will be involved in closing roads, but also in ensuring access for evacuation of casualties without total disruption of the event.

Medical personnel and uniforms

St John Ambulance Brigade and other organisations have their own uniforms and for large participant events the additional medical teams of sports medicine doctors, physiotherapists, and podiatrists must have distinctive clothing, which should be easily visible and practical. It should be possible to distinguish them from each other and from other event staff, who will probably be wearing uniforms emblazoned with sponsors' corporate logos. Sports medicine specialists may work well alongside the first aid organisations or may function better with defined roles separate from the first aiders—for example, staffing a finish medical area while the first aid organisation manages aid points along the route, or running physiotherapy or podiatry tents at the finish. All medical personnel must be accredited and their roles defined beforehand.

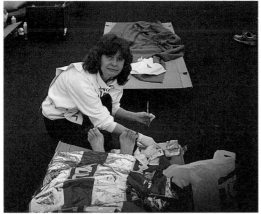

A podiatrist treats the blisters of a London marathon runner at the finish.

Medical advice to marathon, half marathon, and long distance runners*

- Training
- Diet
- Fluids
- Clothing
- What to do on the day
- What to do at the finish
- Medical aid

*Guidelines produced by a consensus conference and published in *BMJ* 1984;**288**:1356-8.

St John Ambulance Brigade staff looking after runners in the first aid tent at the finish of the London marathon.

First aid and casualty management at marathons, half marathons, and long distance runs*

- Hypothermia or exposure
- Hyperthermia, heat stroke, or heat collapse
- Hypovolaemic collapse
- Hypoglycaemia

*Guidelines produced by a consensus conference and published in *BMJ* 1984;**288**:1356-8.

Medical advice to participants

The London marathon sends a medical advice sheet to all participants. It has been widely copied by other events. The emphasis is on the runners taking responsibility for looking after their own health. If they are unwell or injured, or cannot run 15 miles happily one month before the event, they are offered an an inducement not to run—namely, guaranteed entry the following year.

Participants in these gruelling events should be free agents and not under pressure to participate. Raising money for charity removes this freedom, and many mass participation events such as road races have a large number of sponsored runners, often participating to raise money rather than primarily for love of the event. These present a greater risk than the average participants because they may take part despite illness or injury.

There is a trend towards participation by people with various types of medical problem or disability. A marathon run has been claimed as the ultimate goal for those receiving cardiac rehabilitation. Patients with heart and kidney transplants, amputations, diabetes, epilepsy, leukaemia, cancer, asthma, motor neurone disease, multiple sclerosis, and, of course, paraplegia all present potential medical problems. All should appreciate that they take part at their own risk and should receive advice from their own doctors.

Of 25 000 runners in the London marathon each year, some 6 to 16 respond to the request to inform the medical director of any important medical problems they may have, suggesting that there is a large degree of denial of illness among marathon runners. All competitors are encouraged to record any medication they take on the back of their competition number.

Triage and security areas

Access to medical areas should be restricted to casualties and medical staff. Ideally there should be one way in and one way out so that casualties can be "clocked in and out" and relatives, other event staff, and the press do not gain access and get in the way. On arrival each casualty should be triaged. In the London marathon areas are set aside for management of different types of casualty. The more severe constitutional problems such as exercise associated collapse and other constitutional problems, which may require intravenous fluids and a large degree of medical supervision, are treated in the intensive care area. Other areas are set aside for the walking and hopping wounded largely with leg injuries, who often require chiropody or physiotherapy and can sit on chairs. Another is for patients with fatigue and muscle cramps, who respond readily to oral fluids and massage.

INDEX

Index

Index

Index

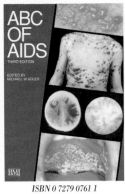
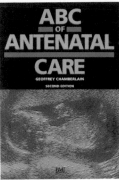
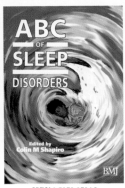
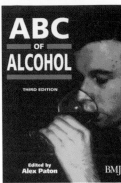
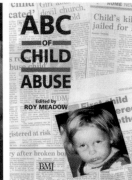
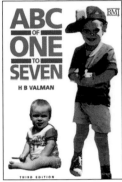
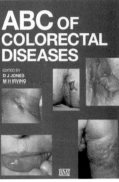
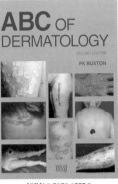
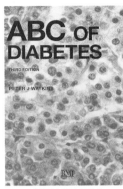
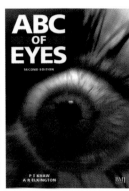
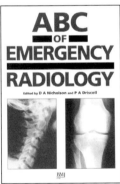
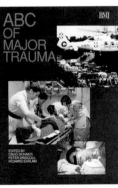
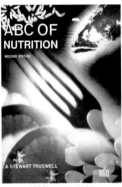
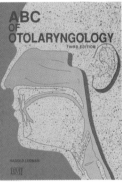
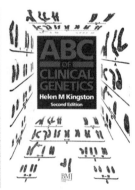
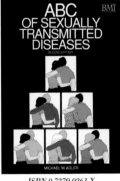
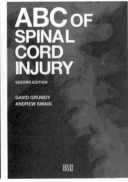
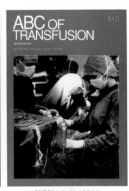
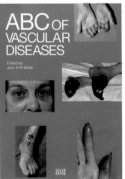
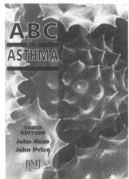
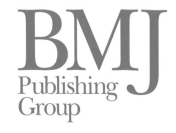